Anshan Gold Standard Mini Atlas Series

HISTOLOGY

Anshan Gold Standard Mini Atlas Series

HISTOLOGY

INDERBIR SINGH
52, Sector One
Rohtak 124001

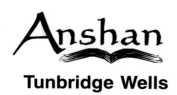

Tunbridge Wells
UK

JAYPEE BROTHERS
MEDICAL PUBLISHERS (P) LTD
New Delhi

First published in the UK by

Anshan Ltd
in 2007
6 Newlands Road
Tunbridge Wells
Kent TN4 9AT, UK

Tel: +44 (0)1892 557767
Fax: +44 (0)1892 530358
E-mail: info@anshan.co.uk
www.anshan.co.uk

ISBN 10   1-905740-30-1
ISBN 13   978-1-905740-30-7

British Library Cataloguing in Publication Data
A catalogue record for this book is available from the British Library

Printed in India by Ajanta Offset & Packagings Ltd., New Delhi

Preface

This small, convenient volume will be useful for rapid revision of the salient features to be seen in histology slides of various tissues of the body.

The book is part of a new Mini Atlas Series being published by the house of Jaypee Brothers Medical Publishers (P) Ltd and Anshan UK.

I am grateful to Shri Jitendar P Vij (CMD) Jaypee Brothers Medical Publishers (P) Ltd. for this initiative, and for his keen interest.

Rohtak   **Inderbir Singh**

Contents

CHAPTER ONE

Epithelia

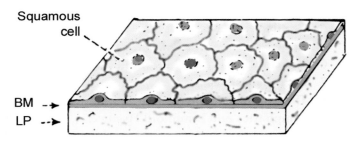

Fig. 1.1. Simple squamous epithelium (diagrammatic).
BM= Basement membrane; LP= Lamina propria.

Squamous Epithelium

The cytoplasm of cells in this kind of epithelium forms only a thin layer. The nuclei produce bulgings of the cell surface. In surface view the cells have polygonal outlines that interlock with those of adjoining cells. With the EM the junctions between cells are marked by occluding junctions: the junctions are thus tightly sealed and any substance passing through the epithelium has to pass through the cells, and not between them.

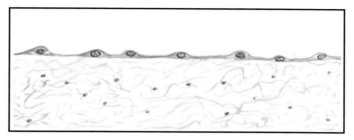

Fig. 1.2. Simple squamous epithelium
as seen in a section.

Squamous epithelium lines the alveoli of the lungs. It lines the free surface of the serous pericardium, of the pleura, and of the peritoneum: here it is called **mesothelium**. It lines the inside of the heart, where it is called **endocardium**; and of blood vessels and lymphatics, where it is called **endothelium**. Squamous epithelium is also found lining some parts of the renal tubules, and in some parts of the internal ear.

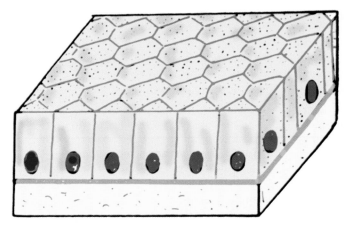

Fig. 1.3. Simple columnar epithelium (diagrammatic). Note the basally placed oval nuclei. The cells appear hexagonal in surface view.

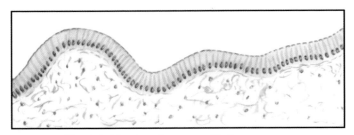

Fig. 1.4. Simple columnar epithelium as seen in a section.

Columnar Epithelium

In vertical section the cells of this epithelium are rectangular. On surface view (or in transverse section) the cells are polygonal. In keeping with the elongated shape of the cells, the nuclei are also frequently elongated.

Columnar epithelium can be further classified according to the nature of the free surfaces of the cells as follows:

(**a**) In some situations the cell surface has no particular specialization: this is *simple columnar epithelium*.

(**b**) In some situations the cell surface bears cilia. This is *ciliated columnar epithelium* (Figs 1.5 and 1.6).

(**c**) In other situations the surface is covered with microvilli. Although the microvilli are visible only with the EM, with the light microscope the region of the microvilli is seen as a *striated border* (when the microvilli are arranged regularly)(Fig. 1.7) or as a *brush border* (when the microvilli are irregularly placed).

Simple columnar epithelium (without cilia or microvilli) is present over the mucous membrane of the stomach and the large intestine.

Columnar epithelium with a striated border is seen most typically in the small intestine, and with a brush border in the gallbladder.

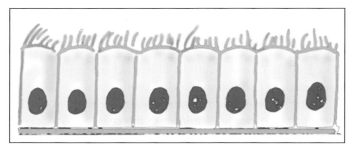

Fig. 1.5. Columnar epithelium showing cilia (diagrammatic).

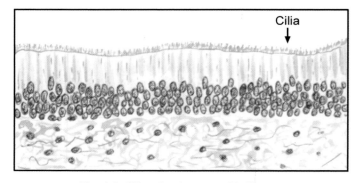

Fig. 1.6. Ciliated columnar epithelium as seen in a section.

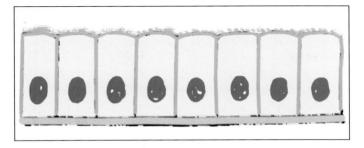

Fig. 1.7. Columnar epithelium showing a striated border made up of microvilli (diagrammatic).

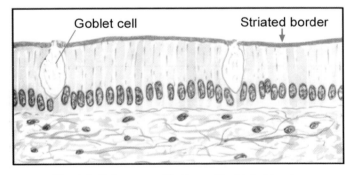

Fig. 1.8. Columnar epithelium with striated border as seen in a section.

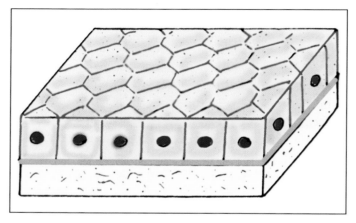

Fig. 1.9. Simple cuboidal epithelium (diagrammatic). Note that the cells appear cuboidal in section and hexagonal in surface view.

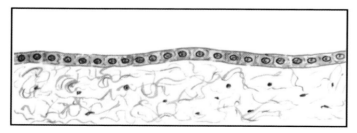

Fig. 1.10. Simple cuboidal epithelium as seen in a section.

Cuboidal Epithelium

Cuboidal epithelium is similar to columnar epithelium, but for the fact that the height of the cells is about the same as their width. The nuclei are usually rounded.

A typical cuboidal epithelium may be seen in the follicles of the thyroid gland, in the ducts of many glands, and on the surface of the ovary (where it is called ***germinal epithelium***). Other sites are the choroid plexuses, the inner surface of the lens, and the pigment cell layer of the retina.

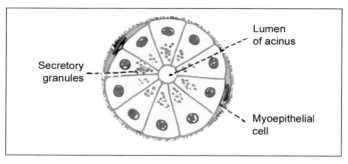

Fig. 1.11. Modified columnar cells in the wall of an acinus (of a gland) (diagrammatic). Note the triangular shape of the cells, the presence of secretory granules, and the myoepithelial cells lying between the gland cells and the basement membrane.

An epithelium that is basically cuboidal (or columnar) lines the secretory elements of many glands. In this situation, however, the parts of the cells nearest the lumen are more compressed (against neighbouring cells) than at their bases, giving them a triangular shape.

A cuboidal epithelium with a prominent brush border is seen in the proximal convoluted tubules of the kidneys.

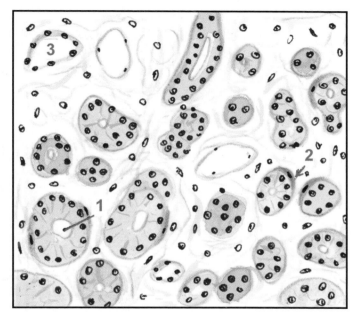

Fig. 1.12. Section through lacrimal gland showing acini of the kind described in Figure 1.11.

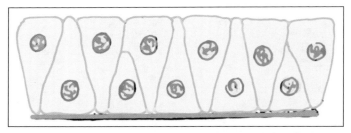

Fig. 1.13. Pseudostratified columnar epithelium (diagrammatic). This figure explains why the nuclei lie at various levels.

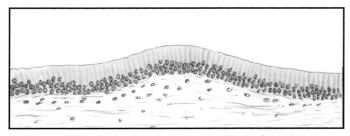

Fig. 1.14. Realistic appearance of pseudostratified columnar epithelium as seen in a section.

Pseudostratified Columnar Epithelium

In usual classroom slides the boundaries between epithelial cells are often not clearly seen. In spite of this we can make out what type of epithelium it is. This is because the shape and spacing of the nuclei gives a good idea of where the cell boundaries must lie.

Normally, in columnar epithelium the nuclei lie in a row, towards the bases of the cells. Sometimes, however, the nuclei appear to be arranged in two or more layers giving the impression that the epithelium is more than one cell thick (Fig. 1.14). The reason for this will be understood easily from Figure 1.13. It is seen that there is actually only one layer of cells, but some cells are broader near the base, and others near the apex. The nuclei lie in the broader part of each cell and are, therefore, not in one layer. To distinguish this kind of epithelium from a true stratified epithelium, it is referred to as ***pseudostratified columnar epithelium***.

A pseudostratified columnar epithelium is found in some parts of the auditory tube, the ductus deferens, and the male urethra (membranous and penile parts). A ciliated pseudostratified columnar epithelium is seen in the trachea and in large bronchi (Fig. 1.6).

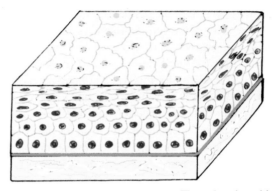

Fig. 1.15. Stratified squamous epithelium. There is a basal layer of columnar cells that rests on the basement membrane. Overlying the columnar cells of this layer there are a few layers of polygonal cells or rounded cells. Still more superficially, the cells undergo progressive flattening, becoming squamous.

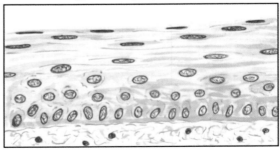

Fig. 1.16. Stratified squamous epithelium (non-keratinized) as seen in a section.

Stratified Squamous Epithelium

This type of epithelium is made up of several layers of cells. The cells of the deepest (or basal) layer rest on the basement membrane: they are usually columnar in shape. Lying over the columnar cells there are polyhedral or cuboidal cells. As we pass towards the surface of the epithelium these cells become progressively more flat, so that the most superficial cells consist of flattened squamous cells (Fig. 1.15).

Stratified squamous epithelium can be divided into two types: ***non-keratinized*** and ***keratinized***. In situations where the surface of the epithelium remains moist, the most superficial cells are living and nuclei can be seen in them. This kind of epithelium is described as non-keratinized. In contrast, at places where the epithelial surface is dry (as in the skin) the most superficial cells die and lose their nuclei. These cells contain a substance called ***keratin***, which forms a non-living covering over the epithelium. This kind of epithelium constitutes keratinized stratified squamous epithelium.

Stratified squamous epithelium (both keratinized and non-keratinized) is found over those surfaces of the body that are subject to friction. As a result of friction the most superficial layers are constantly being removed and are replaced by proliferation of cells from the basal (or germinal) layer. This layer, therefore, shows frequent mitoses.

Keratinized stratified squamous epithelium covers the skin of the whole of the body and forms the epidermis. Non-keratinized stratified squamous epithelium is seen lining the mouth, the tongue, the pharynx, the oesophagus, the vagina and the cornea. Under pathological conditions the epithelium in any of these situations may become keratinized.

Transitional Epithelium (see page 17)

This is a multi-layered epithelium and is 4 to 6 cells thick. It differs from stratified squamous epithelium in that the cells at the surface are not squamous. The deepest cells are columnar or cuboidal. The middle layers are made up of polyhedral or pear-shaped cells. The cells of the surface layer are large and often shaped like an umbrella (Fig. 1.17).

Transitional epithelium is found in the renal pelvis and calyces, the ureter, the urinary bladder, and part of the urethra. Because of this distribution it is also called **urothelium**. In the urinary bladder it is seen that transitional epithelium can be stretched considerably without being damaged. When stretched it appears to be thinner and the cells become flattened or rounded.

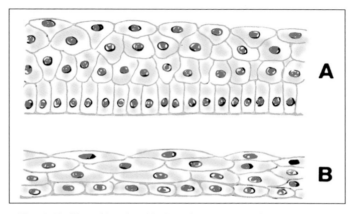

Fig. 1.17. Transitional epithelium (diagrammatic) in unstretched (A), and in stretched, (B) conditions.

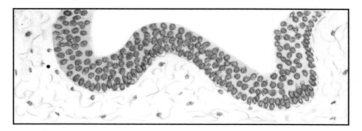

Fig. 1.18. Realistic appearance of transitional epithelium as seen in a section.

CHAPTER TWO

Glands

Some glands are **unicellular**. Most glands are, however, **multicellular**. Such glands develop as diverticulae from epithelial surfaces. The 'distal' parts of the diverticulae develop into secretory elements, while the 'proximal' parts form ducts through which secretions reach the epithelial surface.

When all the secretory cells of an exocrine gland discharge into one duct the gland is said to be a **simple gland**. Sometimes there are a number of groups of secretory cells, each group discharging into its own duct. These ducts unite to form larger ducts which ultimately drain on to an epithelial surface. Such a gland is said to be a **compound gland**.

Both in simple and in compound glands the secretory cells may be arranged in various ways.

(**a**) The secretory element may be **tubular**.

(**b**) The cells may form rounded sacs or **acini**.

(**c**) They may form flask shaped structures called **alveoli**.

(**d**) Combinations of the above may be present in a single gland (as shown on pages 20 and 21).

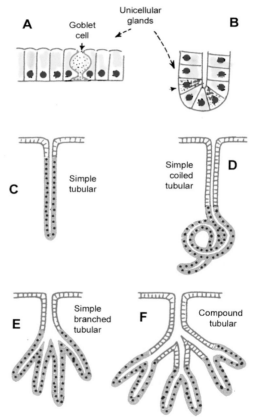

Fig. 2.1A to F (see Legend on page 21).

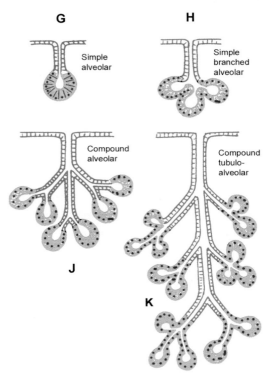

Fig. 2.1A to K. Scheme to show various ways in which the secretory elements of a gland may be organized. A and B are examples of unicellular glands. All others are multicellular. Glands with a single duct are simple glands, while those with a branching duct system are compound glands.

CHAPTER THREE

General Connective Tissue

The term **connective tissue** is applied to a tissue that fills the interstices between more specialized elements; and serves to hold them together and support them.

Connective tissue serves to hold together, and to support, different elements within an organ. Such connective tissue is to be found in almost every part of the body. This kind of connective tissue is referred to as **general connective tissue** is also called **fibro-collagenous tissue**.

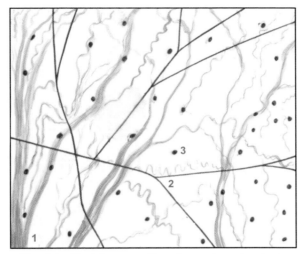

Fig. 3.1. Stretch preparation of omentum showing loose areolar tissue.

Fibres in Connective Tissue

The most conspicuous components of connective tissue are the fibres within it. These are of three main types:

(**a**) **Collagen fibres** are most numerous. They can be classified into various types.

(**b**) **Reticular fibres** were once described as a distinct variety of fibres, but they are now regarded as one variety of collagen fibre.

(**c**) **Elastic fibres**.

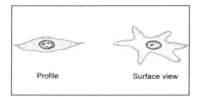

Profile   Surface view

Fig. 3.2. Structure of a fibroblast.

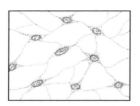

Fig. 3.3. Mesenchymal cells.

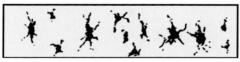

Fig. 3.4. Pigment cells.

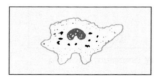

Fig. 3.5. Macrophage cell (histiocyte).

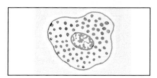

Fig. 3.6. Mast cell.

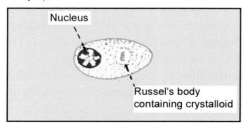

Nucleus

Russel's body containing crystalloid

Fig. 3.7. Plasma cell.

Cells in General Connective Tissue

Various types of cells are present in connective tissue. These can be classed into two distinct categories:

(a) Cells that are intrinsic components of connective tissue: In typical connective tissue the most important cells are *fibroblasts*. Others present are *undifferentiated mesenchymal cells, pigment cells*, and *fat cells*. Other varieties of cells are present in more specialized forms of connective tissues.

(b) Cells that belong to the immune system and are identical or closely related with certain cells present in blood and in lymphoid tissues.

These include *macrophage cells* (or *histiocytes*), *mast cells*, *lymphocytes, plasma cells*, *monocytes* and *eosinophils*.

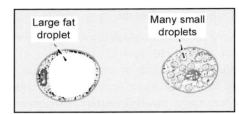

Large fat droplet

Many small droplets

Fig. 3.8. Comparison of a normal fat cell with one in brown fat.

Structure of Adipose Tissue

Adipose tissue is basically an aggregation of fat cells, also called adipocytes. Each fat cell contains a large droplet of fat that almost fills it (Fig. 3.8). As a result the cell becomes rounded. The cytoplasm of the cell forms a thin layer just deep to the plasma membrane. The nucleus is pushed against the plasma membrane and is flattened.

Fat cells can be seen easily by spreading out a small piece of fresh omentum taken from an animal, on a slide. They are best seen in regions where the layer of fat is thin. The fat content can be brightly stained by using certain dyes (Sudan III, Sudan IV) (Fig. 3.10). During the preparation of usual classroom slides, the tissues have to be treated with fat solvents (like xylene or benzene) which dissolve out the fat, so that in such preparations fat cells look like rounded empty spaces (Fig. 3.9). The fat content of the cells can be preserved by cutting sections after freezing the tissue (frozen sections): in this process the tissue is not exposed to fat solvents.

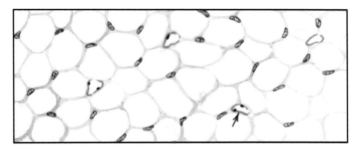

Fig. 3.9. Adipose tissue as seen in a routine paraffin section. The cells look empty as the fat dissolves during processing of tissue.

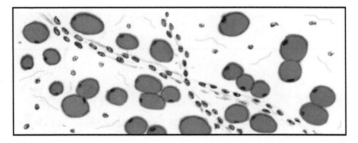

Fig. 3.10. Fat cells in a stretch preparation of omentum stained with a specific stain for fat (Sudan IV).

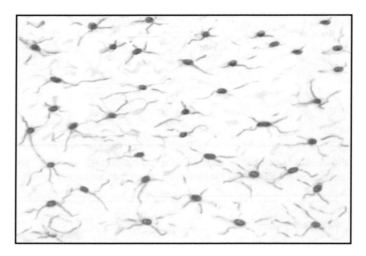

Fig. 3.11. Mucoid tissue.

Mucoid Tissue

In contrast to all the connective tissues described so far the most conspicuous component of mucoid tissue is a jelly like ground substance rich in hyaluronic acid. Scattered through this ground substance there are star-shaped fibroblasts, some delicate collagen fibres and some rounded cells (Fig. 3.11). This kind of tissue is found in the umbilical cord. The vitreous of the eyeball is a similar tissue.

CHAPTER FOUR

Cartilage

Cartilage is considered to be a modified connective tissue. It resembles ordinary connective tissue in that the cells in it are widely separated by a considerable amount of intercellular material or **matrix**. The latter consists of a homogeneous **ground substance** within which fibres are embedded. (Some authorities use the term matrix as an equivalent of ground substance, while others include embedded fibres under the term). Cartilage differs from typical connective tissue mainly in the nature of the ground substance: this is firm and gives cartilage its characteristic consistency. Three main types of cartilage can be recognized depending on the number and variety of fibres in the matrix. These are **hyaline cartilage**, **fibrocartilage** and **elastic cartilage**.

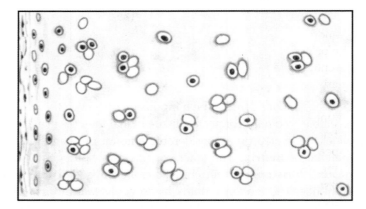

Fig. 4.1. Hyaline cartilage. Note groups of chondrocytes surrounded by homogeneous matrix. Perichondrium is seen at the left end of the figure.

Hyaline Cartilage

Hyaline cartilage is so called because it is transparent (hyalos = glass). Its intercellular substance appears to be homogeneous, but using special techniques it can be shown that many collagen fibres are present in the matrix. In haematoxylin and eosin-stained preparations the matrix is stained blue, i.e. it is basophilic. However, the matrix just under the perichondrium is acidophilic (Fig. 4.1). The structure of the matrix has been described above.

Towards the centre of a mass of hyaline cartilage the chondrocytes are large and are usually present in groups (of two or more). The groups are formed by division of a single parent cell. The cells tend to remain together as the dense matrix prevents their separation. Groups of cartilage cells are called **cell nests** (or **isogenous cell groups**). Immediately around lacunae housing individual chondrocytes, and around cell nests the matrix stains deeper than elsewhere giving the appearance of a capsule. This deep staining matrix is newly formed and is called the **territorial matrix** or **lacunar capsule**. In contrast the pale staining matrix separating cell nests is the **interstitial matrix**. Towards the periphery of the cartilage the cells are small, and elongated in a direction parallel to the surface. Just under the perichondrium the cells become indistinguishable from fibroblasts.

Embedded in the ground substance of hyaline cartilage, there are numerous collagen fibres. The fibres are arranged so that they resist tensional forces. Hyaline cartilage has been compared to a tyre. The ground substance (corresponding to the rubber of the tyre) resists compressive forces, while the fibres (corresponding to the treads of the tyre) resist tensional forces.

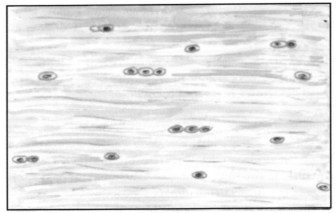

Fig. 4.2. Fibrocartilage. Cartilage cells are embedded amongst thick bundles of collagen fibres.

Fibrocartilage

On superficial examination this type of cartilage (also called **white fibrocartilage**) looks very much like dense fibrous tissue (Fig. 4.2). However, in sections it is seen to be cartilage because it contains typical cartilage cells surrounded by capsules. The matrix is pervaded by numerous collagen bundles amongst which there are some fibroblasts.

The fibres merge with those of surrounding connective tissue, there being no perichondrium over the cartilage. This kind of cartilage has great tensile strength combined with considerable elasticity.

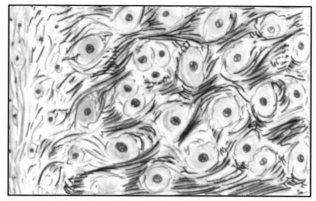

Fig. 4.3. Elastic cartilage. Note chondrocytes surrounded by bundles of elastic fibres. The section has been stained by Verheoff's method in which elastic fibres are stained bluish-black.

Elastic Cartilage

Elastic cartilage (or yellow fibrocartilage) is similar in many ways to hyaline cartilage. The main difference is that instead of collagen fibres, the matrix contains numerous elastic fibres that form a network (Fig. 4.3). The fibres are difficult to see in haematoxylin and eosin-stained sections, but they can be clearly visualized if special methods for staining elastic fibres are used. The surface of elastic cartilage is covered by perichondrium.

Elastic cartilage possesses greater flexibility than hyaline cartilage, and readily recovers its shape after being deformed.

CHAPTER FIVE

Bone

Some Features of Gross Structure

If we examine a longitudinal section across a bone (such as the humerus) we see that the wall of the shaft is tubular and encloses a large **marrow cavity**. The wall of the tube is made up of a hard dense material that appears, on naked eye examination, to have a uniform smooth texture with no obvious spaces in it. This kind of bone is called **compact bone**. It is seen further, that compact bone is thickest midway between the two ends of the bone and gradually tapers towards the ends.

When we examine the bone ends we find that the marrow cavity does not extend into them. They are filled by a meshwork of tiny rods or plates of bone and contain numerous spaces, the whole appearance resembling that of a sponge. This kind of bone is called **spongy** or **cancellous bone** (cancel= cavity). The spongy bone at the bone ends is covered by a thin layer of compact bone, thus providing the bone ends with smooth surfaces. Small bits of spongy bone are also present over the wall of the marrow cavity.

Where the bone ends take part in forming joints they are covered by a layer of articular cartilage. With the exception of the areas covered by articular cartilage, the entire outer surface of bone is covered by a membrane called the **periosteum**. The wall of the marrow cavity is lined by a membrane called the **endosteum**.

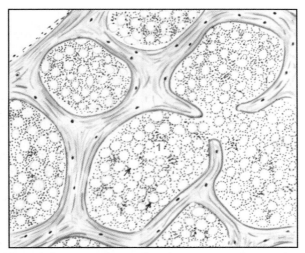

Fig. 5.1. Structure of cancellous bone as seen in a section.
1-Bone marrow.

Structure of Cancellous Bone

The bony plates or rods that form the meshwork of cancellous bone are called **trabeculae**. Each trabeculus is made up of a number of lamellae (described above) between which there are lacunae containing osteocytes. Canaliculi, containing the processes of osteocytes, radiate from the lacunae.

The trabeculae enclose wide spaces that are filled in by bone marrow. They receive nutrition from blood vessels in the bone marrow (Fig. 5.1).

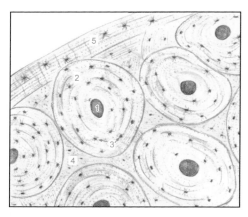

Fig. 5.2. Structure of compact bone as seen in a ground section. 1= Haversian canal. 2=Concentric lamellae forming Haversian system. 3= Lacunae. 4. Interstitial lamellae. 5. Circumferential lamellae.

Structure of Compact Bone

When we examine a section of compact bone we find that this type of bone is also made up of lamellae, and is pervaded by lacunae (containing osteocytes), and by canaliculi. Most of the lamellae are arranged in the form of concentric rings that surround a narrow ***Haversian canal*** present at the centre of each ring. The Haversian canal is occupied by blood vessels, nerve fibres, and some cells. One Haversian canal and the lamellae around it constitute a ***Haversian system*** or ***osteon***.

When we examine longitudinal sections through compact bone we find that the Haversian canals (and, therefore, the osteons) run predominantly along the length of the bone. The canals branch and anastomose with each other. They also communicate with the marrow cavity, and with the external surface of the bone through channels that are called the **canals of Volkmann**. Blood vessels and nerves pass through all these channels so that compact bone is permeated by a network of blood vessels that provide nutrition to it.

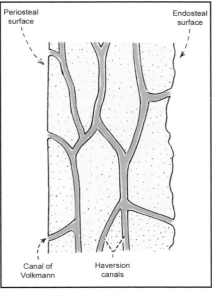

Fig. 5.3. Schematic longitudinal section through compact bone to show Haversian canals and the canals of Volkmann.

Osteoblasts

These are bone forming cells. They are found lining growing surfaces of bone.

The nucleus of an osteoblast is ovoid and euchromatic. The cytoplasm is basophilic because of the presence of abundant rough endoplasmic reticulum.

Osteoblasts are responsible for laying down the organic matrix of bone including the collagen fibres. They are also responsible for calcification of the matrix.

Osteoclasts

These are bone removing cells. They are found in relation to surfaces where bone removal is taking place. (Bone removal is essential for maintaining the proper shape of growing bone).

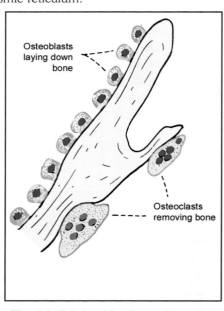

Osteoblasts laying down bone

Osteoclasts removing bone

Fig. 5.4. Relationship of osteoblasts and osteoclasts to developing bone.

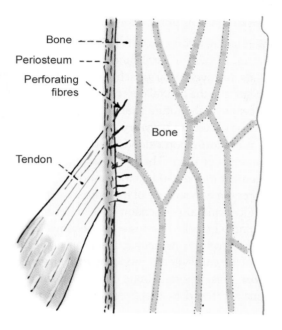

Fig. 5.5. Diagram to show the perforating fibres (of Sharpey).

The periosteum provides a medium through which muscles, tendons and ligaments are attached to bone. In situations where very firm attachment of a tendon to bone is necessary, the fibres of the tendon continue into the outer layers of bone as the ***perforating fibres of Sharpey***.

Development of a Typical Long Bone

In the region where a long bone is to be formed the mesenchyme first lays down a cartilaginous model of the bone. This cartilage is covered by perichondrium. Endochondral ossification starts in the central part of the cartilaginous model (i.e. at the centre of the future shaft).

This area is called the **primary centre of ossification**. Gradually, bone formation extends from the primary centre towards the ends of shaft. This is accompanied by progressive enlargement of the cartilaginous model.

Soon after the appearance of the primary centre, and the onset of endochondral ossification in it, the perichondrium (which may now be called periosteum) becomes active. The osteoprogenitor cells in its deeper layer lay down bone on the surface of the cartilaginous model by **intramembranous ossification**. This periosteal bone completely surrounds the cartilaginous shaft and is, therefore, called the **periosteal collar**.

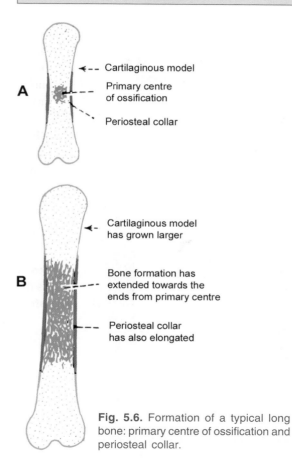

A

- Cartilaginous model
- Primary centre of ossification
- Periosteal collar

B

- Cartilaginous model has grown larger
- Bone formation has extended towards the ends from primary centre
- Periosteal collar has also elongated

Fig. 5.6. Formation of a typical long bone: primary centre of ossification and periosteal collar.

The periosteal collar is first formed only around the region of the primary centre, but rapidly extends towards the ends of the cartilaginous model (Fig. 5.6B). It acts as a splint, and gives strength to the cartilaginous model at the site where it is weakened by the formation of secondary areolae. We shall see that most of the shaft of the bone is derived from this periosteal collar and is, therefore, membranous in origin.

At about the time of birth the developing bone consists of (a) a part called the **diaphysis** (or shaft), that is bony, and has been formed by extension of the primary centre of ossification, and (b) ends that are cartilaginous (Fig.5.7A).

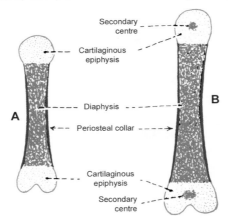

Fig. 5.7. Formation of a typical long bone: secondary centres of ossification.

At varying times after birth **secondary centres** of endochondral ossification appear in the cartilages forming the ends of the bone (Fig. 5.7B). These centres enlarge until the ends become bony (Fig. 5.8). More than one secondary centre of ossification may appear at either end. The portion of bone formed from one secondary centre is called an **epiphysis**.

For a considerable time after birth the bone of the diaphysis and the bone of any epiphysis are separated by a plate of cartilage called the **epiphyseal cartilage**, or **epiphyseal plate**. This is formed by cartilage into which ossification has not extended either from the diaphysis or from the epiphysis. We shall see that this plate plays a vital role in growth of the bone.

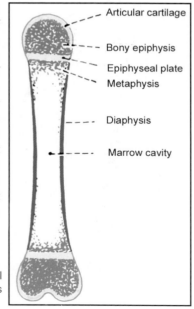

Articular cartilage

Bony epiphysis

Epiphyseal plate

Metaphysis

Diaphysis

Marrow cavity

Fig. 5.8. Formation of a typical long bone: bony epiphyses and epiphyseal plates.

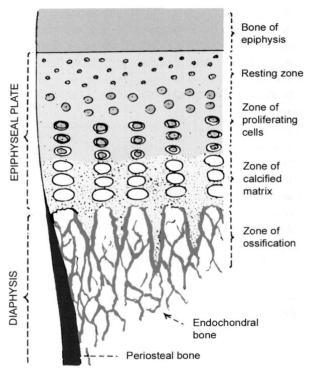

Fig. 5.9. Structure of an epiphyseal plate.

To understand how a bone grows in length, we will now take a closer look at the epiphyseal plate. Depending on the arrangement of cells, three zones can be recognized (Fig. 5.9).

(**a**) *Zone of resting cartilage*: Here the cells are small and irregularly arranged.

(**b**) *Zone of proliferating cartilage*: This is also called the *zone of cartilage growth*. In this zone the cells are larger, and undergo repeated mitosis. As they multiply, they come to be arranged in parallel columns, separated by bars of intercellular matrix.

(**c**) *Zone of calcification*: This is also called the *zone of cartilage transformation*. In this zone the cells become still larger and the matrix becomes calcified.

Next to the zone of calcification, there is a zone where cartilage cells are dead and the calcified matrix is being replaced by bone. Growth in length of the bone takes place by continuous transformation of the epiphyseal cartilage to bone in this zone (i.e. on the diaphyseal surface of the epiphyseal cartilage).

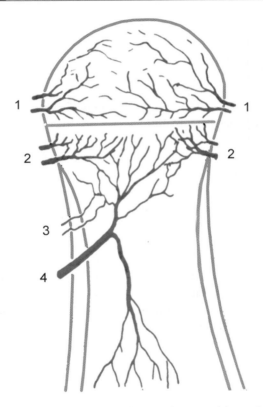

Fig. 5.10. Scheme to show the arteries supplying a long bone. 1-epiphyseal; 2-metaphyseal; 3-periosteal; 4-nutrient. The veins (not shown) accompany the arteries.

A long bone receives three sets of arteries:

1. A **nutrient artery** (or more accurately a **diaphyseal nutrient artery**) pierces the shaft near its middle and enters the marrow cavity. Sometimes more than one nutrient artery may be present. The opening for the nutrient artery is called the **nutrient foramen**. The foramen leads into a canal that passes obliquely through the shaft. The canal is directed away from the growing end of the bone (i.e. the end where the epiphysis fuses with the shaft later than at the other end). Within the marrow cavity the artery divides into ascending and descending branches.

2. Several arteries enter the bone near either end. Some of these are **epiphyseal arteries**, while others are **metaphyseal arteries**.

3. Several small arteries arise from periosteal vessels and enter the bone through minute foramina (Fig. 5.10).

Branches of all these arteries form a rich sinusoidal plexus in bone marrow. Many branches from the plexus enter Haversian canals through communications of the latter with the marrow cavity. Periosteal arteries reach the Haversian canals through the canals of Volkmann.

CHAPTER SIX

Muscle

Muscle tissue is composed predominantly of cells that are specialized to shorten in length by contraction. This contraction results in movement. It is in this way that virtually all movements within the body, or of the body in relation to the environment, are ultimately produced.

Muscle tissue is made up basically of cells that are called **myocytes**. Myocytes are elongated in one direction and are, therefore, often referred to as **muscle fibres**. We shall see, however, that in some cases muscle fibres are made up of several myocytes joined to each other; or of greatly elongated myocytes containing multiple nuclei.

Skeletal muscle is made up essentially of long, cylindrical 'fibres'. The length of the fibres is highly variable, the longest being as much as 30 cm in length. The diameter of the fibres also varies considerably (10-60 μm: usually 50-60 μm). Each 'fibre' is really a syncytium with hundreds of nuclei along its length. (The 'fibre' is formed, during development, by fusion of numerous myoblasts). The nuclei are elongated and lie along the periphery of the fibre, just under the cell membrane (which is called the **sarcolemma**). The cytoplasm (or **sarcoplasm**) is filled with numerous longitudinal fibrils that are called **myofibrils**.

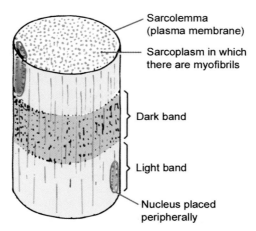

Sarcolemma (plasma membrane)

Sarcoplasm in which there are myofibrils

Dark band

Light band

Nucleus placed peripherally

Fig. 6.1. Scheme to show the structure of a muscle fibre.

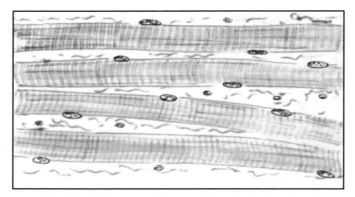

Fig. 6.2. Skeletal muscle seen in longitudinal section.

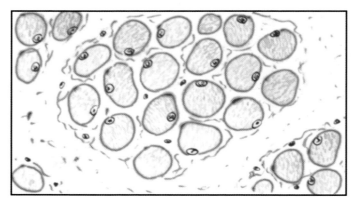

Fig. 6.3. Skeletal muscle seen in transverse section.

The most striking feature of skeletal muscle fibres is the presence of transverse striations in them. After staining with haematoxylin the striations are seen as alternate dark and light bands that stretch across the muscle fibre. The dark bands are called **A-bands**, while the light bands are called **I-bands**. (As an aid to memory note that 'A' and 'I' correspond to the second letters in the words d**a**rk and l**i**ght.

In good preparations (specially if the fibres are stretched) some further details can be made out. Running across the middle of each I-band there is a thin dark line called the **Z-band**. The middle of the A-band is traversed by a lighter band, called the **H-band** (or **H-zone**). Running through the centre of the H-band a thin dark line can be made out. This is the **M-band**.

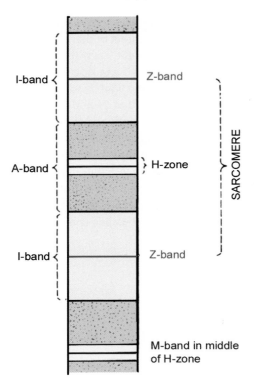

Fig. 6.4. Scheme to show the terminology of transverse bands in a myofibril. Note that the A-band is confined to one sarcomere, but the I-band is made up of parts of two sarcomeres that meet at the Z-band.

Connective Tissue Framework of Muscles

Muscles are pervaded by a network of connective tissue fibres. This connective tissue supports muscle fibres and unites them to each other. Individual muscle fibres are surrounded by delicate connective tissue that is called the **endomysium**. Individual fasciculi are surrounded by a stronger sheath of connective tissue called the **perimysium**. Connective tissue that surrounds the entire muscle is called the **epimysium**. At the junction of a muscle with a tendon the fibres of the endomysium, the perimysium and the epimysium become continuous with the fibres of the tendon.

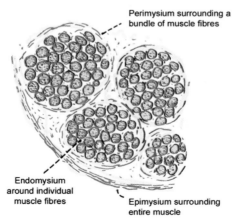

Perimysium surrounding a bundle of muscle fibres

Endomysium around individual muscle fibres

Epimysium surrounding entire muscle

Fig. 6.5. Diagram to show the connective tissue present in relation to skeletal muscle.

The structure of cardiac muscle has many similarities to that of skeletal muscle; but there are important differences as well.

These are follows. Like skeletal muscle, cardiac muscle is made up of elongated 'fibres' within which there are numerous myofibrils. The myofibrils (and, therefore, the fibres) show transverse striations similar to those of skeletal muscle. A, I, Z and H bands can be made out in the striations. The connective tissue framework, and the capillary network around cardiac muscle fibres are similar to those in skeletal muscle.

1. The fibres of cardiac muscle do not run in strict parallel formation, but branch and anastomose with other fibres to form a network.

2. Each fibre of cardiac muscle is not a multinucleated syncytium as in skeletal muscle, but is a chain of cardiac muscle cells (or ***cardiac myocytes***) each having its own nucleus. Each myocyte is about 80 μm long and about 15 μm broad.

3. The nucleus of each myocyte is located centrally (and not peripherally as in skeletal muscle).

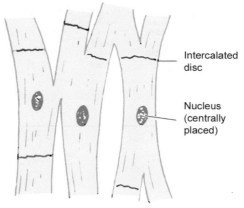

Intercalated
disc

Nucleus
(centrally
placed)

Fig. 6.6. Cardiac muscle (diagrammatic).
Also see Figure 6.7.

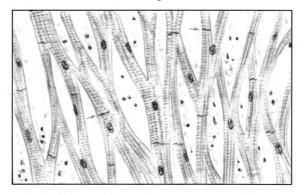

Fig. 6.7. Cardiac muscle as seen in a section.

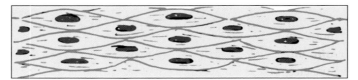

Fig. 6.8. Smooth muscle cells (diagrammatic).

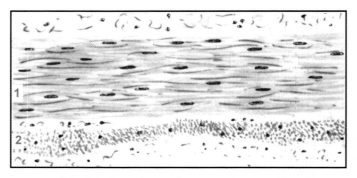

Fig. 6.9. Smooth muscle as seen in a section.
1-L.S. 2-T.S.

Basic Facts About Smooth Muscle

Smooth muscle (also called ***non-striated, involuntary*** or ***plain muscle***) is made up of long spindle shaped cells (myocytes) having a broad central part and tapering ends. The nucleus, which is oval or elongated, lies in the central part of the cell. The length of smooth muscle cells (often called fibres) is highly variable (15 μm to 500 μm).

With the light microscope the sarcoplasm appears to have indistinct longitudinal striations, but there are no transverse striations.

Smooth muscle cells are usually aggregated to form bundles, or fasciculi, that are further aggregated to form layers of variable thickness. In such a layer the cells are so arranged that the thick central part of one cell is opposite the thin tapering ends of adjoining cells. Aggregations of smooth muscle cells into fasciculi and layers is facilitated by the fact that each myocyte is surrounded by a network of delicate fibres (collagen, reticular, elastic) that holds the myocytes together. The fibres between individual myocytes become continuous with the more abundant connective tissue that separates fasciculi or layers of smooth muscle.

CHAPTER SEVEN

Nervous Tissue

A neuron consists of a **cell body** that gives off a variable number of **processes**. The cell body is also called the **soma** or **perikaryon**. Like a typical cell it consists of a mass of cytoplasm surrounded by a cell membrane. The cytoplasm contains a large central nucleus (usually with a prominent nucleolus), numerous mitochondria, lysosomes and a Golgi complex.

The processes arising from the cell body of a neuron are called **neurites.** These are of two kinds. Most neurons give

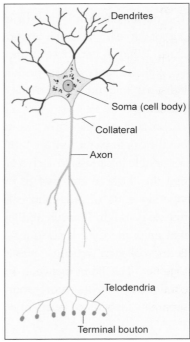

Fig. 7.1. Scheme to show some parts of a neuron.

off a number of short branching processes called **dendrites**
and one longer process called an **axon.**

The cytoplasm shows the presence of a granular material
that stains intensely with basic dyes; this material is the **Nissl
substance** (also called Nissl bodies or granules) (Fig. 7.2).
When examined by EM, these bodies are seen to be composed
of rough surfaced endoplasmic reticulum.

The presence of abundant granular endoplasmic reticulum
is an indication of the high level of protein synthesis in neurons.
The proteins are needed for maintenance and repair, and for
production of neurotransmitters and enzymes.

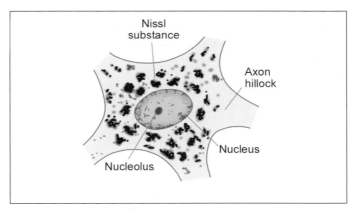

Fig. 7.2. Neuron stained to show Nissl substance. Note that the
Nissl substance extends into the dendrites but not into the axon.

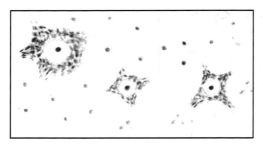

Fig. 7.3. Section of spinal cord showing large neurons in the ventral grey column.

Another distinctive feature of neurons is the presence of a network of fibrils permeating the cytoplasm (Fig. 7.4). These **neurofibrils** are seen, with the EM, to consist of microfilaments and microtubules.

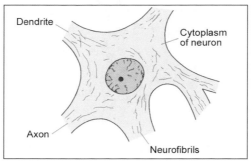

Fig. 7.4. Neuron stained to show neurofibrils. Note that the fibrils extend into both axons and dendrites.

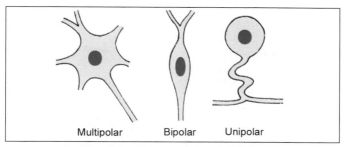

Multipolar   Bipolar   Unipolar

Fig. 7.5. Diagram showing three types of neurons.

Variation in the Shape of Neuronal Cell Bodies

Neurons vary considerably in the size and shape of their cell bodies (somata) and in the length and manner of branching of their processes. The cell body varies in diameter from about 5 μm, in the smallest neurons, to as much as 120 μm in the largest ones. The shape of the cell body is dependent on the number of processes arising from it. The most common type of neuron gives off several processes and the cell body is, therefore, **multipolar**. Some neurons have only one axon and one dendrite and are **bipolar.**

Another type of neuron has a single process (which is highly convoluted). After a very short course this process divides into two. One of the divisions represents the axon; the other is functionally a dendrite, but its structure is indistinguishable from that of an axon. This neuron is described as **unipolar**, but from a functional point of view it is to be regarded as bipolar. Depending on the shapes of their cell bodies some neurons are referred to as **stellate** (star shaped) or **pyramidal.**

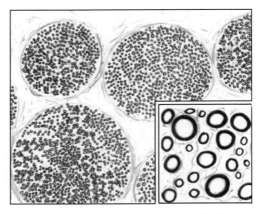

Fig. 7.6. Section through peripheral nerve stained by a method in which the myelin sheaths become black. The inset shows fibres at high magnification.

Each nerve fibre has a central core formed by the axon. This core is called the ***axis cylinder***. The plasma membrane surrounding the axis cylinder is the ***axolemma***. The axis cylinder is surrounded by a myelin sheath. This sheath is in the form of short segments that are separated at short intervals called the ***nodes of Ranvier***. The part of the nerve fibre between two consecutive nodes is the ***internode.*** Each segment of the myelin sheath is formed by one Schwann cell. Outside the myelin sheath there is a thin layer of Schwann cell cytoplasm. This layer of cytoplasm is called the ***neuri-lemma.***

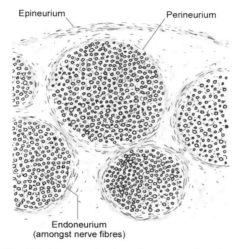

Epineurium   Perineurium

Endoneurium
(amongst nerve fibres)

Fig. 7.7. Diagram to show the connective tissue
supporting nerve fibres in a peripheral nerve.

Each nerve fibre is surrounded by a layer of connective
tissue called the ***endoneurium*** (Fig. 7.7). The endoneurium
holds adjoining nerve fibres together and facilitates their
aggregation to form bundles or ***fasciculi***. Apart from collagen
fibres the endoneurium contains fibroblasts, Schwann cells,
endothelial cells and macrophages.

Each fasciculus is surrounded by a thicker layer of
connective tissue called the ***perineurium***. The perineurium
is made up of layers of flattened cells separated by layers of
collagen fibres. The perineurium probably controls diffusion
of substances in and out of axons.

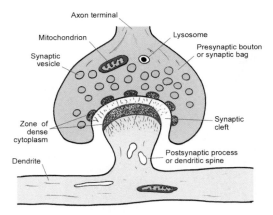

Fig. 7.8. Scheme showing the structure of a
typical synapse as seen by EM.

Synapses are sites of junction between neurons. Synapses
may be of various types depending upon the parts of the
neurons that come in contact. In the most common type of
synapse, an axon terminal establishes contact with the
dendrite of a receiving neuron to form an **axodendritic
synapse.**

A synapse transmits an impulse only in one direction. The
two elements taking part in a synapse can, therefore, be
spoken of as **presynaptic** and **postsynaptic** (Fig. 7.8). In
an axo-dendritic synapse, the terminal enlargement of the
axon may be referred to as the **presynaptic bouton** or
synaptic bag. The region of the dendrite receiving the axon
terminal is the **postsynaptic process**. The two are separated
by a space called the **synaptic cleft.**

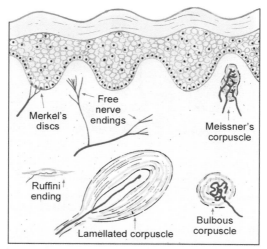

Fig. 7.9. Some sensory receptors present in relation to skin.

Tactile Corpuscles (of Meissner)

These are small oval or cylindrical structures seen in relation to dermal papillae in the hand and foot, and in some other situations. These corpuscles are believed to be responsible for touch.

Pacinian corpuscles are circular or oval structures. These are much larger than tactile corpuscles. Lamellated corpuscles respond to pressure and vibration.

Bulbous Corpuscles (of Krause)

These are spherical structures about 50 μm in diameter.

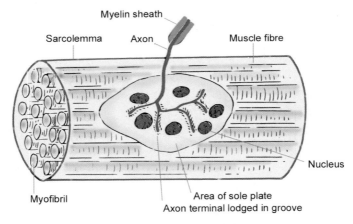

Fig. 7.10. Motor end plate seen in relation to a muscle fibre (surface view). Schwann cell cytoplasm covering the nerve terminal has not been shown for sake of clarity.

Each skeletal muscle fibre receives its own direct innervation. The site where the nerve ending comes into intimate contact with the muscle fibre is a ***neuromuscular (or myoneural) junction***.

In most neuromuscular junctions the nerve terminal comes in contact with a specialized area near the middle of the muscle fibre. This area is roughly oval or circular, and is referred to as the ***sole plate***. The sole plate plus the axon terminal constitute the ***motor end plate***.

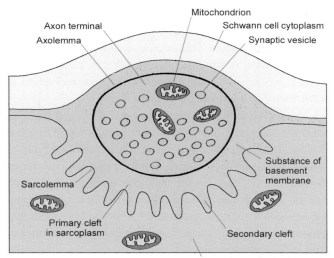

Fig. 7.11. Neuromuscular junction. This figure is a section across one of the axon terminals (and related structures) shown in Fig. 7.10. These details are seen only by EM.

Structure of a Typical Motor End Plate

In the region of the motor end plate axon terminals are lodged in grooves in the sarcolemma covering the sole plate. Between the axolemma (over the axon) and the sarcolemma (over the muscle fibre) there is a narrow gap (about 40 nm) occupied by various proteins that form a basal lamina. It follows that there is no continuity between axoplasm and sarcoplasm.

Axon terminals are lodged in grooves in the sarcolemma covering the sole plate. In section this groove is seen as a semicircular depression. This depression is the ***primary cleft.*** The sarcolemma in the floor of the primary cleft is thrown into numerous small folds resulting in the formation of ***secondary (or subneural) clefts.***

In the region of the sole plate the sarcoplasm of the muscle fibre is granular. It contains a number of nuclei and is rich in mitochondria, endoplasmic reticulum and Golgi complexes.

Axon terminals are also rich in mitochondria. Each terminal contains vesicles similar to those seen in presynaptic boutons. The vesicles contain the neurotransmitter acetylcholine. Acetylcholine is released when nerve impulses reach the neuromuscular junction. It initiates a wave of depolarisation in the sarcolemma resulting in contraction of the entire muscle fibre. Thereafter the acetylcholine is quickly destroyed by the enzyme acetyl choline esterase. The presence of acetylcholine receptors has been demonstrated in the sarcolemma of the sole plate.

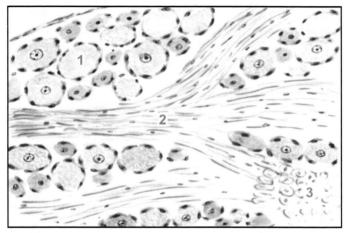

Fig. 7.12. Section through a sensory ganglion. Note large neurons arranged in groups separated by bundles of nerve fibres.

Structure of Sensory Ganglia

In haematoxylin and eosin stained sections the neurons of sensory ganglia are seen to be large and arranged in groups chiefly at the periphery of the ganglion (Fig. 7.12). The groups of cells are separated by groups of myelinated nerve fibres.

The entire ganglion is pervaded by fine connective tissue. The ganglion is covered on the outside by a connective tissue capsule.

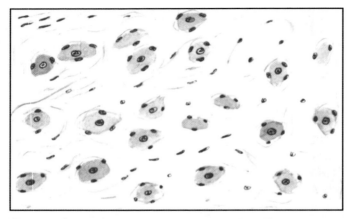

Fig. 7.13. Section through an autonomic ganglion. The neurons are not arranged in groups but are scattered amongst nerve fibres.

Structure of Autonomic Ganglia

The neurons of autonomic ganglia are smaller than those in sensory ganglia (Fig. 7.13). With silver impregnation they are seen to be multipolar. The neurons are not arranged in definite groups as in sensory ganglia, but are scattered throughout the ganglion. The nerve fibres are non-myelinated and thinner. They are, therefore, much less conspicuous than in sensory ganglia.

CHAPTER EIGHT
The Cardiovascular System

The cardiovascular system consists of the heart and of blood vessels. The blood vessels that take blood from the heart to various tissues are called *arteries*. The smallest arteries are called *arterioles*. Arterioles open into a network of *capillaries* that pervade the tissues. Exchanges of various substances between the blood and the tissues take place through the walls of capillaries. In some situations, capillaries are replaced by slightly different vessels called *sinusoids*. Blood from capillaries (or from sinusoids) is collected by small *venules* that join to form *veins*. The veins return blood to the heart.

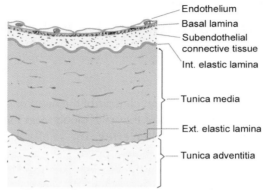

Fig. 8.1. Scheme to show the layers in
the wall of a typical artery.

Arteries

The wall of an artery is made up of three layers.

(**1**) The innermost layer is called the ***tunica intima*** (tunica
= coat). It consists of (**a**) an endothelial lining; (**b**) a thin
layer called the ***basal lamina***; (**c**) a delicate layer of
subendothelial connective tissue; and (**d**) of a membrane
formed by elastic fibres called the ***internal elastic lamina***.

(**2**) Outside the tunica intima there is the ***tunica media*** or
middle layer. The media may consist predominantly of elastic
tissue or of smooth muscle. On the outside the media is limited
by a membrane formed by elastic fibres: this is the external
elastic lamina.

(**3**) The outermost layer is called the ***tunica adventitia***.

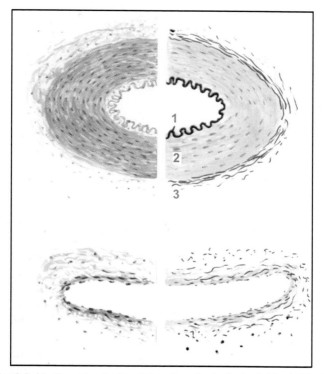

Fig. 8.2. Medium sized artery (above) and vein (below). The left half of the figure shows the appearance as seen with haematoxylin and eosin staining. The right half shows appearance when elastic fibres are stained black (Verhoeff's method). 1-Internal elastic lamina. 2-Tunica media. 3-Tunica adventitia

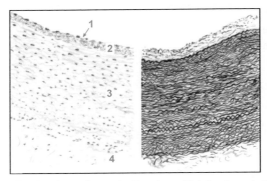

Fig. 8.3. Section through an elastic artery. Staining is as in Fig. 8.2. 1-Endothelial lining. 2-Tunica intima. 3-Tunica media. 4-Tunica adventitia.

Elastic and Muscular Arteries

On the basis of the kind of tissue that predominates in the tunica media, arteries are often divided into elastic arteries and muscular arteries. Elastic arteries include the aorta and the large arteries supplying the head and neck (carotids) and limbs (subclavian, axillary, iliac). The remaining arteries are muscular.

Although all arteries carry blood to peripheral tissues, elastic and muscular arteries play differing additional roles. When the left ventricle of the heart contracts, and blood enters the large elastic arteries with considerable force, these arteries distend significantly. They are able to do so because of much elastic tissue in their walls. During diastole (i.e., relaxation of the left ventricle) the walls of the arteries come back to their original size because of the elastic recoil of their walls. This recoil acts as an additional force that pushes the blood into smaller arteries. It is because of this fact that blood flows continuously through arteries (but with fluctuation of pressure during systole and diastole). In contrast a muscular artery has the ability to alter the size of its lumen by contraction or relaxation of smooth muscle in its wall. Muscular arteries can, therefore, regulate the amount of blood flowing into the regions supplied by them.

Details of the differences in structure of elastic and muscular arteries are given below.

Differences between Elastic and Muscular Arteries

The main difference in structure of elastic and muscular arteries is in the constitution of the tunica media. In elastic arteries the media is made up mainly of elastic tissue. The elastic tissue is in the form of a series of concentric membranes. In the aorta (which is the largest elastic artery) there may be as many as fifty layers of elastic membranes. On the contrary in muscular arteries the media is made up mainly of smooth muscle. This muscle is arranged circularly.

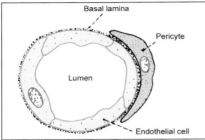

Fig. 8.4. Diagram to show the structure of a continuous capillary.

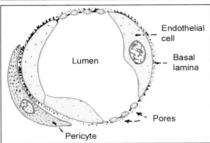

Fig. 8.5. Diagram to show the structure of a fenestrated capillary.

Terminal exchanges (of oxygen, carbon dioxide, fluids and various molecules) between blood and tissue take place through the walls of the capillary plexus. The average diameter of a capillary is 8 μm. The wall of a capillary is formed essentially by endothelial cells that are lined on the outside by a basal lamina (glycoprotein). Overlying the basal lamina there may be isolated branching perivascular cells (pericytes), and a delicate network of reticular fibres and cells.

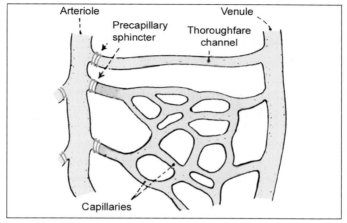

Fig. 8.6. Diagram to show precapillary sphincters and thoroughfare channels.

Precapillary Sphincters and Thoroughfare Channels

Arteriovenous anastomoses described above control blood flow through relatively large segments of the capillary bed. Much smaller segments can be individually controlled as follows.

Capillaries arise as side branches of terminal arterioles. The initial segment of each such branch is surrounded by a few smooth muscle cells that constitute a ***precapillary sphincter***. Blood flow, through any part of the capillary bed, can be controlled by the precapillary sphincter.

In many situations, arterioles and venules are connected (apart from capillaries) by some channels that resemble capillaries, but have a larger calibre. These channels run a relatively direct course between the arteriole and venule. Isolated smooth muscle fibres may be present on their walls. These are called ***thoroughfare channels***. At times when most of the precapillary sphincters in the region are contracted (restricting flow through capillaries), blood is short circuited from arteriole to venule through the thoroughfare channels. A thoroughfare channel and the capillaries associated with it are sometimes referred to as a ***microcirculatory unit***.

CHAPTER NINE

Lymphatics and Lymphoid Tissue

Lymphoid tissues are those in which there are prominent aggregations of lymphocytes. These include lymph nodes which are small bean-shaped structures present in various parts of the body. A fluid called lymph reaches these nodes from tissues through lymphatic vessels. Lymphatic vessels interconnect the lymph nodes. Ultimately lymph reaches large lymphatic ducts and is poured into veins.

Other lymphatic organs are the thymus, the spleen and the tonsils. Aggregations of lymphocytes are also seen in the walls of the gut, the trachea and bronchi.

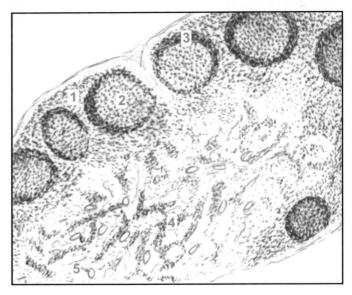

Fig. 9.1. Section through a lymph node. 1-Cortex. 2, 3-Germinal center and outer zone of lymphatic follicle. 4-Medulla. 5-Blood vessel.

Lymph Node

Each lymph node consists of a connective tissue framework; and of numerous lymphocytes. The entire node is bean-shaped. The node has an outer zone that contains densely packed lymphocytes, and therefore stains darkly: this part is the **cortex**. Surrounded by the cortex, there is a lighter staining zone in which lymphocytes are fewer: this area is the **medulla**. Within the cortex there are several rounded areas that are called **lymphatic follicles** or **lymphatic nodules**. Each nodule has a paler staining **germinal centre** surrounded by a zone of densely packed lymphocytes.

Within the medulla the lymphocytes are arranged in the form of anastomosing cords. Several blood vessels can be seen in the medulla.

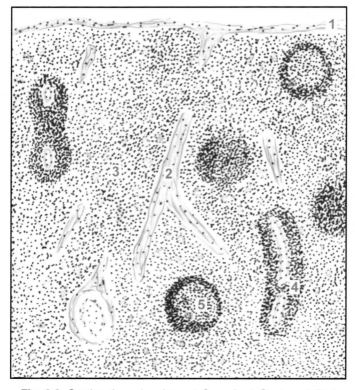

Fig. 9.2. Section through spleen. 1-Capsule. 2-Septum. 3-Red pulp. 4, 5-Cords of densely packed lymphocytes around arteriole.

Spleen

This section is stained by haematoxylin and eosin. Note the capsule (1) and the septa or trabeculae (2) extending into the organ from the capsule. The substance of the organ is divisible into the red pulp (3) in which there are diffusely distributed lymphocytes and numerous sinusoids; and the white pulp in which dense aggregations of lymphocytes are present. The latter are in the form of cords surrounding arterioles (4). When cut transversely (5) the cords resemble the lymphatic nodules of lymph nodes, and like them they have germinal centres surrounded by rings of densely packed lymphocytes. However, the nodules of the spleen are easily distinguished from those of lymph nodes because of the presence of an arteriole in each nodule. The arteriole is placed eccentrically at the margin of the germinal centre.

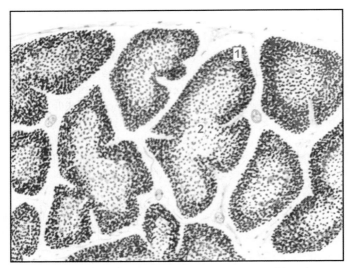

Fig. 9.3. Thymus (low power view). Note masses of lymphocytes arranged in the form of lobules. 1-Cortex. 2-Medulla. 3-Hassal's corpuscle.

Thymus

This organ is made up of lymphoid tissue arranged in the form of distinct lobules. The presence of this lobulation enables easy distinction of the thymus from all other lymphoid organs. The lobules are partially separated from each other by connective tissue. Each lobule has an outer cortex (1) in which

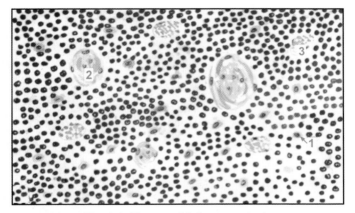

Fig. 9.4. Thymus. (High power view).
1- Epithelial cell. 2-Hassall's corpuscle. 3-Capillary.

lymphocytes are densely packed; and an inner medulla (2)
in which the cells are diffuse. The medulla contains pink
staining rounded masses called the corpuscles of Hassall (3).
In this figure the corpuscles are seen as pink staining rounded
masses. Their central parts appear homogeneous, but the
peripheral parts are made up of concentrically arranged cells.
In this figure also note the diffusely distributed lymphocytes.
Scattered amongst them there are cells with a pink staining
cytoplasm: these are epithelial cells. Some blood capillaries
are also seen.

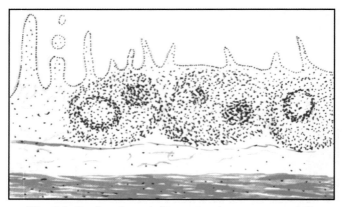

Fig. 9.5. Section through ileum showing an aggregated lymphatic follicle (Peyer's patch) in the submucosa.

Mucosa Associated Lymphoid Tissue in the Alimentary System

This is also called **gut associated lymphoid tissue** (GALT).

Small collections of lymphoid tissue, similar in structure to the follicles of lymph nodes, may be present anywhere along the length of the gut. They are called **solitary lymphatic follicles**. Larger aggregations of lymphoid tissue, each consisting of 10 to 200 follicles are also present in the small intestine. They are called **aggregated lymphatic follicles** or **Peyer's patches**. These patches can be seen by naked eye, and about 200 of them can be counted in the human gut.

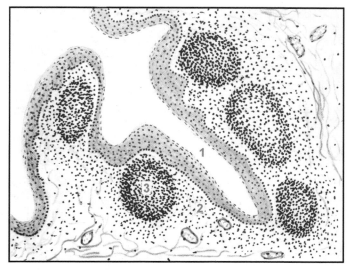

Fig. 9.6. Section through palatine tonsil. 1-Crypt. 2-Diffuse lymphoid tissue. 3- Lymphatic nodule.

Palatine Tonsil

This is an aggregation of lymphoid tissue that is readily recognized by the fact that it is covered by a stratified squamous epithelium. At places the epithelium dips into the tonsil in the form of deep crypts (1). Deep to the epithelium there is diffuse lymphoid tissue (2) in which typical lymphatic nodules (3) can be seen.

CHAPTER TEN

Skin and its Appendages

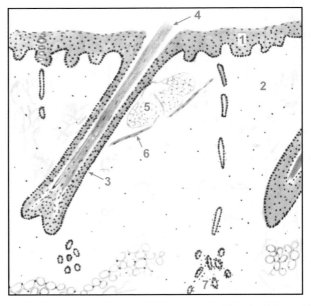

Fig. 10.1. Section through skin. 1-Epidermis. 2-Dermis. 3-Hair follicle. 4-Hair. 5-Sebaceous gland. 6- Arrector pili. 7-Sweat gland.

Skin

In Figure 10.1 we see a low power view of the skin. Note the epidermis (1), the dermis (2), a hair follicle (3) with a hair (4) in it, a sebaceous gland (5), an arrector pili muscle (6) and parts of sweat glands (7). Some adipose tissue is present in the deeper part. Each sebaceous gland consists of a number of alveoli that open into a hair follicle. Each alveolus is pear shaped. It consists mainly of a solid mass of polyhedral cells.

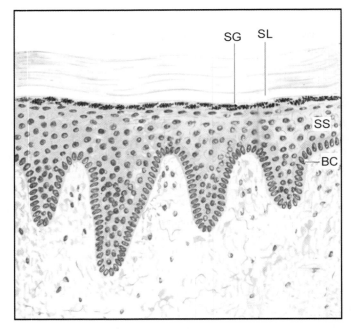

Fig. 10.2. Section through skin showing the layers of the epidermis. SC-Stratum corneum. SL-Stratum lucidum. SG-Stratum granulosum. SS-Stratum spinosum. BC-Basal cell layer.

Epidermis

The epidermis consists of stratified epithelium in which the following layers can be recognized.

(**a**) The deepest or ***basal layer*** (***stratum basale***) is made up of a single layer of columnar cells that rest on a basal lamina.

The basal layer is, therefore, also called the ***germinal layer*** (***stratum germinativum***).

(**b**) Above the basal layer there are several layers of polygonal keratinocytes that constitute the ***stratum spinosum*** (or ***Malpighian layer***).

(**c**) Overlying the stratum spinosum there are a few (1 to 5) layers of flattened cells. These cells constitute the ***stratum granulosum***.

(**d**) Superficial to the stratum granulosum there is the ***stratum lucidum***

(**e**) The most superficial layer of the epidermis is called the ***stratum corneum***. It is made up of flattened scale-like elements (squames)

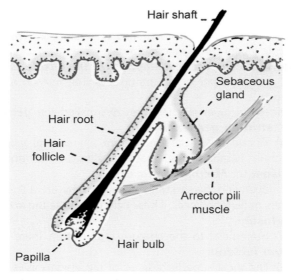

Fig. 10.3. Basic structure of a hair follicle.
Also see Figure 10.1.

Hair Follicle

The hair follicle may be regarded as a part of the epidermis
that has been invaginated into the dermis around the hair
root. Its innermost layer, that immediately surrounds the hair
root is, therefore, continuous with the surface of the skin;
while the outermost layer of the follicle is continuous with
the dermis. Also see pages 93 and 94.

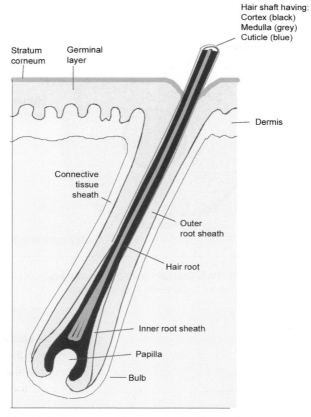

Fig. 10.4. Scheme to show some details of a hair follicle.

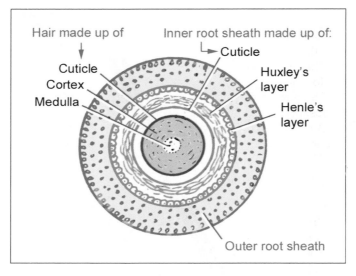

Fig. 10.5. Diagram to show the various
layers to be seen in a hair follicle.

Hair Follicle

The wall of the follicle consists of three main layers. Beginning with the innermost layer they are:

(**a**) The ***inner root sheath*** present only in the lower part of the follicle.

(**b**) The ***outer root sheath*** that is continuous with the stratum spinosum.

(**c**) A connective tissue sheath derived from the dermis.

The inner root sheath is further divisible into the following.

(**1**) The innermost layer is called the ***cuticle***. It lies against the cuticle of the hair, and consists of flattened cornified cells.

(**2**) Next there are one to three layers of flattened nucleated cells that constitute ***Huxley's layer***, or the ***stratum epitheliale granuloferum***. Cells of this layer contain large eosinophilic granules (***trichohyaline granules***).

(**3**) The outer layer (of the inner root sheath) is made up of a single layer of cubical cells with flattened nuclei. This is called ***Henle's layer***, or the ***stratum epitheliale pallidum***.

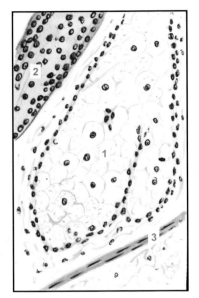

Fig. 10.6. Sebaceous gland (high power view).
1-Sebaceous gland. 2-Part of hair follicle. 3-Arrector pili.

Sebaceous Glands

Sebaceous glands are seen most typically in relation to hair follicles. Each gland consists of a number of alveoli that are connected to a broad duct that opens into a hair follicle. Each alveolus is pear shaped. It consists of a solid mass of poly-hedral cells and has hardly any lumen. The outermost cells are small and rest on a basement membrane. The inner cells are larger, more rounded, and filled with lipid. This lipid is discharged by disintegration of the innermost cells that are replaced by proliferation of outer cells. The sebaceous glands are, therefore, examples of holocrine glands. The secretion of sebaceous glands is called **sebum**. Its oily nature helps to keep the skin and hair soft. It helps to prevent dryness of the skin and also makes it resistant to moisture. Sebum contains various lipids including triglycerides, cholesterol, cholesterol esters and fatty acids.

In some situations sebaceous glands occur independently of hair follicles. Such glands open directly on the skin surface. They are found around the lips, and in relation to some parts of the male and female external genitalia. The tarsal (Meibomian) glands of the eyelid are modified sebaceous glands. Montgomery's tubercles present in the skin around the nipple (areola) are also sebaceous glands. Secretion by sebaceous glands is not under nervous control.

Sweat Glands

Sweat glands produce sweat or perspiration. They are present in the skin over most of the body. Apart from typical sweat glands there are atypical ones present at some sites.

The entire sweat gland consists of a single long tube. The lower end of the tube is highly coiled on itself and forms the **body** (or **fundus**) or the gland. The body is made up of the secretory part of the gland. It lies in the

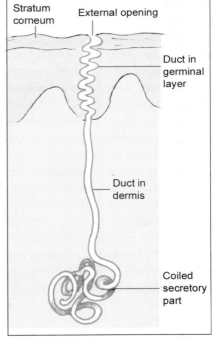

Fig. 10.7. Diagrammatic representation of the parts of a typical sweat gland.

reticular layer of the dermis, or some-times in subcutaneous tissue. The part of the tube connecting the secretory element to the skin surface is the **duct**. It runs upwards through the dermis to reach the epidermis. Within the epidermis the duct follows a spiral course to reach the skin surface. The orifice is funnel shaped. On the palms, soles and digits the openings of sweat glands lie in rows on epidermal ridges.

The wall of the tube making up the gland consists of an inner epithelial lining, its basal lamina, and a supporting layer of connective tissue.

In the secretory part the epithelium is made up of a single layer of cubical or polygonal cells. Sometimes the epithelium may appear to be pseudostratified).

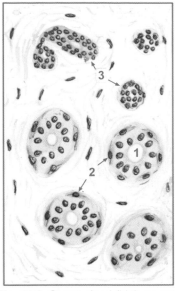

Fig. 10.8. Sweat gland (high power view). 1-Sections through secretory part. 2-Sections through duct.

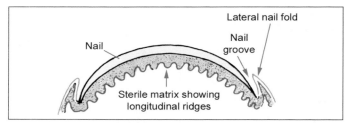

Fig. 10.9. Transverse section across a nail.

Nails

Nails are present on fingers and toes. The main part of a nail is called its **body**. The body has a free distal edge. The proximal part of the nail is implanted into a groove on the skin and is called the **root** (or **radix**). The tissue on which the nail rests is called the **nail bed**. The nail bed is highly vascular, and that is why the nails look pink in colour.

The nail represents a modified part of the zone of keratinization of the epidermis. It is usually regarded as a much thickened continuation of the stratum lucidum, but it is more like the stratum corneum in structure. The nail substance consists of several layers of dead, cornified, 'cells' filled with keratin.

The greater part of each lateral margin of the nail is also overlapped by a skin fold called the **lateral nail fold**. The groove between the lateral nail fold and the nail bed (in which the lateral margin of the nail lies) is called the **lateral nail groove**.

CHAPTER ELEVEN
Respiratory System

The respiratory system consists of the lungs, and the passages through which air reaches them. These passages are the nasal cavities, the pharynx, the trachea, the bronchi and their intrapulmonary continuations. With regard to the pharynx, it should be noted that this organ consists of nasal, oral and laryngeal parts. The nasal part is purely respiratory in function, but the oral and laryngeal parts are more intimately concerned with the alimentary system.

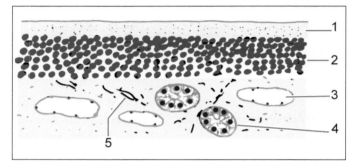

Fig. 11.1. Olfactory mucosa seen in section stained by routine methods. 1. Clear zone of cytoplasm. 2. Several layers of nuclei. 3. Capillary. 4. Bowman's gland. 5. Nerve fibre.

Olfactory Mucosa

This is yellow in colour, in contrast to the pink colour of the respiratory mucosa. It consists of a lining epithelium and a lamina propria.

The ***olfactory epithelium*** is pseudostratified. It is much thicker than the epithelium lining the respiratory mucosa (about 100 μm). Within the epithelium there is a superficial zone of clear cytoplasm below which there are several rows of nuclei. Using special methods three types of cells can be recognized in the epithelium).

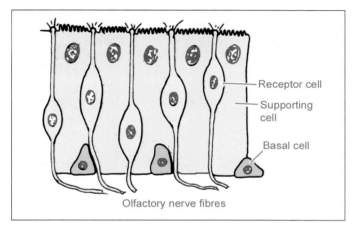

Fig. 11.2. Cells to be seen in olfactory epithelium. RC- receptor cell. SC- supporting cell. BC-basal cell.

(**1**) The *olfactory cells* are modified neurons.

(**2**) The *sustentacular cells* support the olfactory cells. Their nuclei are oval, and lie near the free surface of the epithelium.

(**3**) The *basal cells* lie deep in the epithelium and do not reach the luminal surface. They divide to form new olfactory cells to replace those that die. Some basal cells have a supporting function.

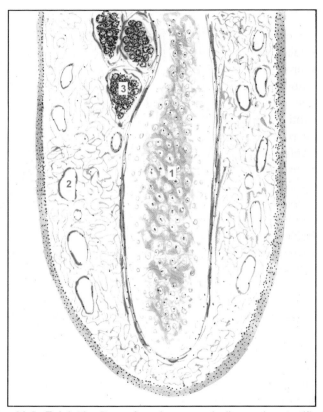

Fig. 11.3. Epiglottis. Its surface is covered all over by stratified squamous epithelium. 1-Elastic cartilage. 2-Blood vessels. 3-Glands.

The Epiglottis

The epiglottis is important because sections through it are usually included in sets of class slides. The epiglottis has a central core of elastic cartilage. Overlying the cartilage there is mucous membrane. The greater part of the mucous membrane is lined by stratified squamous epithelium (non-keratinizing). The mucous membrane over the lower part of the posterior surface of the epiglottis is lined by pseudo-stratified ciliated columnar epithelium. This part of the epiglottis does not come in contact with swallowed food as it is overlapped by the aryepiglottic folds. Some taste buds are present in the epithelium of the epiglottis (A few taste buds may be seen in the epithelium elsewhere in the larynx).

Numerous glands, predominantly mucous, are present in the mucosa deep to the epithelium. Some of them lie in depressions present on the epiglottic cartilage.

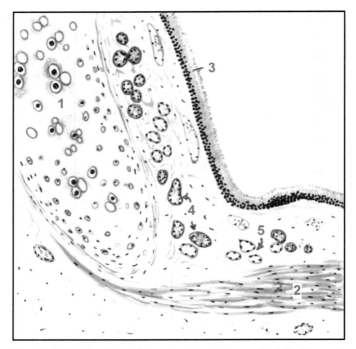

Fig. 11.4. Section through trachea (posterior part). 1-Cartilage. 2-Smooth muscle. 3-Mucous membrane lined by pseudostratified columnar epithelium. 4-Serous gland. 5-Mucous gland.

Trachea

The skeletal basis of the trachea is made up of 16 to 20 tracheal cartilages. Each of these is a C-shaped mass of hyaline cartilage. The gaps between the cartilage ends, present on the posterior aspect, are filled in by smooth muscle and fibrous tissue.

The lumen of the trachea is lined by mucous membrane that consists of a lining epithelium and an underlying layer of connective tissue. The lining epithelium is pseudostratified ciliated columnar. It contains numerous goblet cells, and basal cells that lie next to the basement membrane. Numerous lymphocytes are seen in deeper parts of the epithelium.

The subepithelial connective tissue contains numerous elastic fibres. It contains serous glands that keep the epithelium moist; and mucous glands that provide a covering of mucous in which dust particles get caught. The mucous is continuously moved towards the larynx by ciliary action. Numerous aggregations of lymphoid tissue are present in the subepithelial connective tissue. Eosinophil leucocytes are also present.

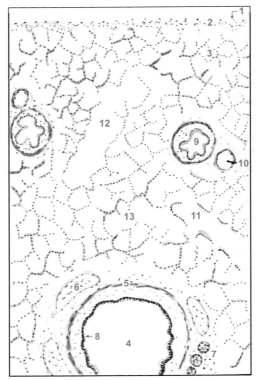

Fig. 11.5. Section through part of a lung. 1, 2-Pleura. 3-Alveolus. 4-Bronchus. 5-Smooth muscle. 6-Cartilage. 7-Glands. 8-Epithelium of bronchus.9-Bronchiole. 10-Artery. 11-Respiratory bronchiole. 12-Alveolar duct. 13-Atrium.

Lung

The lung surface is covered by pleura which consists of a lining of mesothelium (1) resting on a layer of connective tissue (2).

The lung substance is made up of numerous thin-walled spaces or alveoli (3). The alveoli are filled with air that reaches them through a series of respiratory passages some of which are as follows.

A large bronchus (4) is seen in the lower part of the figure. Its structure is similar to that of the trachea in that smooth muscle (5), cartilage (6), and glands (7) are present in its wall; and it is lined by a similar epithelium (8). Two smaller, bronchioles (9) are seen: they are lined by a simple columnar epithelium, and have a wall of smooth muscle. There is no cartilage in their walls. Two arteries (10) are seen near the bronchioles. A respiratory bronchiole is seen at '11', an alveolar duct at '12', and an atrium at '13'.

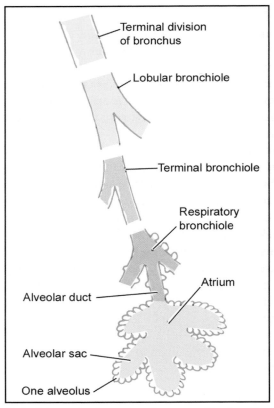

Fig. 11.6. Scheme to show some terms used to describe the terminal ramifications of the bronchial tree.

Intrapulmonary Passages

On entering the lung the principal bronchus divides into secondary, or **lobar bronchi** (one for each lobe). Each lobar bronchus divides into tertiary, or **segmental bronchi** (one for each segment of the lobe). (For precise details of the pattern of segmental bronchi consult a book on gross anatomy). The segmental bronchi divide into smaller and smaller bronchi, which ultimately end in **bronchioles**. The lung substance is divided into numerous lobules each of which receives a **lobular bronchiole**. The lobular bronchiole gives off a number of **terminal bronchioles**. As indicated by their name the terminal bronchioles represent the most distal parts of the conducting passage. Each terminal bronchiole ends by dividing into **respiratory bronchioles**. These are so called because they are partly respiratory in function as some air sacs (see below) arise from them. Each respiratory bronchiole ends by dividing into a few **alveolar ducts**. Each alveolar duct ends in a passage, the **atrium**, which leads into a number of rounded **alveolar sacs**. Each alveolar sac is studded with a number of air sacs or **alveoli**. The alveoli are blind sacs having very thin walls through which oxygen passes from air into blood, and carbon dioxide passes from blood into air.

CHAPTER TWELVE

Oral Cavity and Related Structures

Lip

The substance of the lip is occupied by a mass of skeletal muscle (cut transversely) and by connective tissue. The outer surface (1) of the lip is covered by true skin in which hair follicles (2) and sebaceous glands (3) can be made out. The inner surface is covered by mucous membrane which has a covering of thick stratified squamous epithelium (4), with deep papillae (5) extending into the underlying connective tissue. Numerous glands (6), some serous and some mucous, are present deep to the mucosa. The junction of skin and mucosa lies at (7).

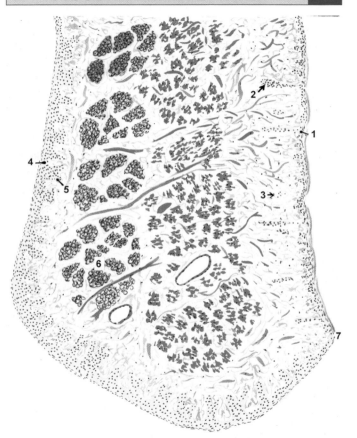

Fig. 12.1. Section through a lip.

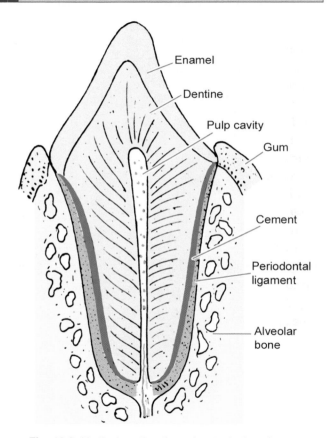

Fig. 12.2. Vertical section through a typical tooth.

Tooth

A tooth consists of an 'upper' part, the **crown**, which is seen in the mouth; and of one or more **roots** which are embedded in sockets in the jaw bone (mandible or maxilla). The greater part of the tooth is formed by a bone-like material called **dentine**. In the region of the crown the dentine is covered by a much harder white material called the **enamel**. Over the root the dentine is covered by a thin layer of **cement**. The cement is united to the wall of the bony socket in the jaw by a layer of fibrous tissue that is called the **periodontal ligament**. The external surface of the alveolar process is covered by the gum that normally overlaps the lower edge of the crown. Within the dentine there is a **pulp canal** (or **pulp cavity**) that contains a mass of cells, blood vessels, and nerves that constitute the **pulp**. The blood vessels and nerves enter the pulp canal through the **apical foramen** which is located at the apex of the root .

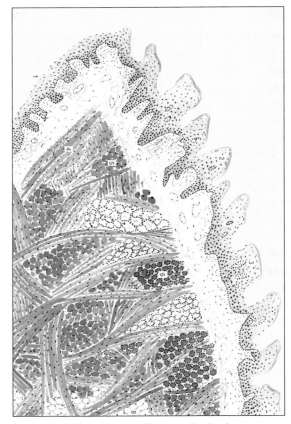

Fig. 12.3. Tongue (Panoramic view).

Tongue

Figure 12.3 is a panoramic view of a section of the tongue near its tip. The surface is covered by stratified squamous epithelium. The undersurface of the tongue is smooth (1), but on the dorsum the surface shows numerous projections or papillae. Each papilla has a core of connective tissue covered by epithelium. Some papillae are pointed (filiform - 2), while others are broad at the top (fungiform - 3). A third type of papilla (circumvallate) is shown in Figure 12.4. The top of this papilla is broad and lies at the same level as the surrounding mucosa. Going right round the papilla there is a deep groove (1). Taste buds (2) are present on both walls of the groove.

The main mass of the tongue is formed by skeletal muscle: The fibres run in various directions so that some are cut longitudinally (4) and some transversely (5). Some of the muscle fibres extend into the circumvallate papillae (4 in Fig. 12.4). Some adipose tissue is present amongst the muscle fibres (8). Numerous serous glands (6) and mucous glands (7) are present amongst the muscle fibres. In Figure 12.4 note the serous glands of Von Ebner (3) opening into the bottom of the sulcus around the circumvallate papilla.

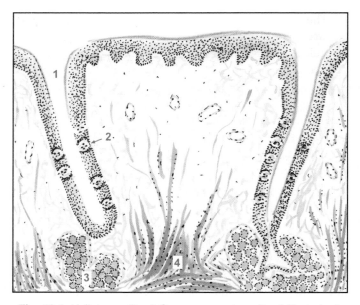

Fig. 12.4. Vallate papilla. 1-Groove around papilla. 2-Taste bud. 3- Serous glands of Von Ebner). 4-Muscle extending into papilla.

The largest papillae of the tongue are called ***circumvallate papillae***. They are arranged in a row just anterior to the sulcus terminalis. When viewed from the surface each papilla is seen to have a circular top demarcated from the rest of the mucosa by a groove. In sections through the papilla it is seen that the papilla has a circumferential 'lateral wall' that lies in the depth of the groove. Taste buds are present on this wall, and also on the 'outer' wall of the groove.

Other papillae present on the tongue are:

(a) Filiform papillae

(b) Fungiform papillae

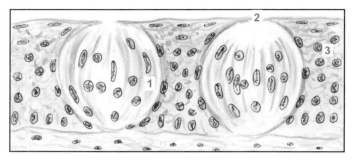

Fig. 12.5. Taste buds. 1-Elongated cells. 2-Pore.
3-Stratified squamous epithelium.

Taste Buds

Taste buds are present in relation to circumvallate papillae,
to fungiform papillae, and to leaf-like folds of mucosa (***folia
linguae***) present on the posterolateral part of the tongue.
Taste buds are also present on the soft palate, the epiglottis,
the palatoglossal arches, and the posterior wall of the oro-
pharynx.

Each taste bud is a piriform structure made up of modified epithelial cells. It extends through the entire thickness of
the epithelium. Each bud has a small cavity that opens to the
surface through a ***gustatory pore***. The cavity is filled by a
material rich in polysaccharides.

The cells present in taste buds are elongated and are
vertically orientated, those towards the periphery being curved

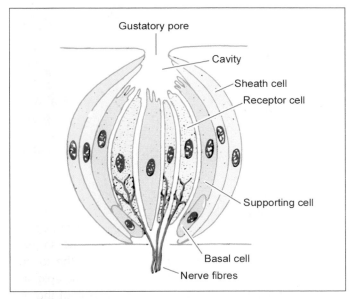

Fig. 12.6. Scheme to show the cells in a taste bud.

like crescents. Each cell has a central broader part containing the nucleus, and tapering ends. The cells are of two basic types. Some of them are **receptor cells** or **gustatory cells**. Endings of afferent nerves end in relation to them. Other cells perform a supporting function.

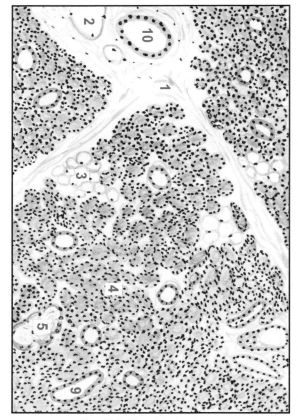

Fig. 12.7. Parotid gland.

Parotid Gland

In Figure 12.7 we see a section through the parotid gland. Compare it with Figure 12.8, which shows a section through the submandibular gland, and with Figure 12.9, which shows a sublingual gland. All these are compound tubulo-alveolar glands. The gland is divided into lobules separated by interlobular connective tissue (1) in which some blood vessels (2) and adipose tissue (3) are present. The glandular tissue is made up of acini. Numerous intralobular (9) and interlobular (10) ducts can be seen.

In the parotid gland (Fig. 12.7) the acini are almost entirely serous (4), but a rare mucous acinus (5) may be seen.

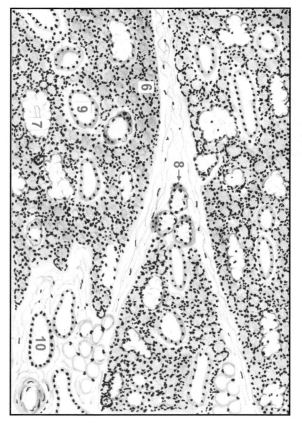

Fig. 12.8. Submandibular gland (low power view).

Submandibular Gland

In general the submandibular gland is similar to the parotid gland. However, both serous (6) and mucous (7) acini are seen. In some cases serous cells are present in relation to mucous acini forming demilunes (or crescents) (8).

In Figure 12.8 we see a high power view of the submandibular gland to show the appearance of serous (1) and mucous (2) acini, and demilunes (3). A duct is also seen (4). Note the myoepithelial cells (5) present in relation to the acini.

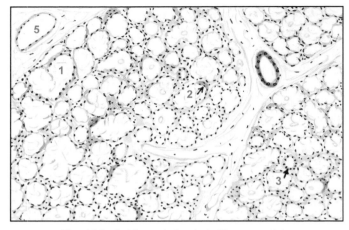

Fig. 12.9. Sublingual gland. 1- Mucous acini.
2-Demilune. 3-Duct.

Sublingual Gland

The general description of this gland is the same as given for the parotid and submandibular glands, but the acini are almost entirely mucous (1). An occasional serous demilune (2) may be seen. Intralobular ducts (3) are relatively few. An interlobular duct is seen at '4', and a blood vessel at '5'.

CHAPTER THIRTEEN

Oesophagus, Stomach and Intestines

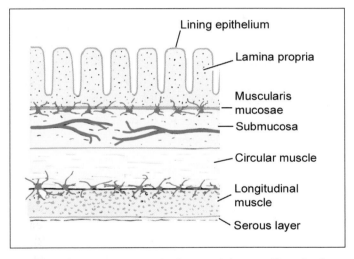

Fig. 13.1. Scheme to show the layers of the gut. Note the large blood vessels in the submucosa; the myenteric nerve plexus between the longitudinal and circular layers of muscle; and the subcutaneous nerve plexus near the muscularis mucosae.

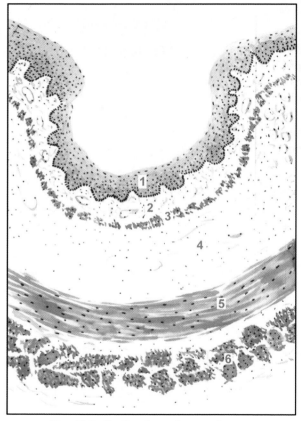

Fig. 13.2. Section through oesophagus.

Oesophagus (T.S)

Note the lining of non-keratinized stratified squamous epithelium (1), the underlying connective tissue of the lamina propria (2), the muscularis mucosae (3) in which the muscle fibres are cut transversely, the submucosa (4), the layer of circular muscle (5), and the layer of longitudinal muscle (6).

The muscle is of the striated variety in the upper one third of the oesophagus, mixed in the middle one third, and smooth in the lower one third.

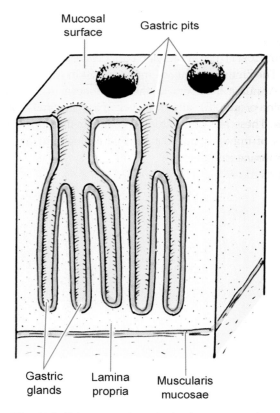

Fig. 13.3. Scheme to show the basic structure of the mucous membrane of the stomach.

The Stomach

The wall of the stomach has the mucous membrane, a submucosa, a muscularis externa, and a serous layer.

The lining epithelium is columnar and mucous secreting.

At numerous places the lining epithelium dips into the lamina propria to form the walls of depressions called ***gastric pits***. These pits extend for a variable distance into the thickness of the mucosa. Deep to the gastric pits the mucous membrane is packed with numerous ***gastric glands***. These glands are of three types: main gastric, cardiac and pyloric.

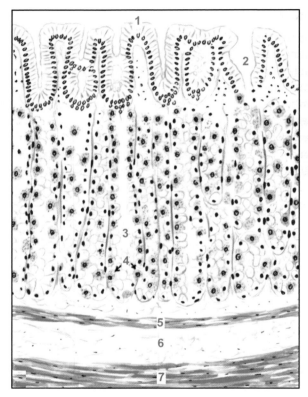

Fig. 13.4. Section through body of the stomach. 1-Lining by columnar epithelium. 2-Gastric pit. 3-Gastric glands. 4-Oxyntic cells. 5-Muscularis mucosae. 6-Submucosa. 7-Circular muscle.

Stomach, Body

Note the thick mucosa, muscularis mucosae (5), submucosa (6) and part of circular muscle coat (7). The mucosa has a lining of columnar epithelium (1) which dips inwards to form numerous gastric pits (2) which occupy the superficial one fourth of the mucosa. The area between the pits and the muscularis mucosae is packed with tubular gastric glands (3). The glands are lined mainly by blue staining chief cells (3) or peptic cells. Amongst these there are pink staining oxyntic cells (4). These are large cells that are placed peripherally in the wall of the gland. They are more numerous in the upper parts of the gastric glands.

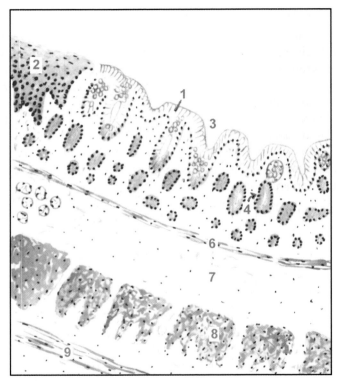

Fig. 13.5. Stomach, cardiac end. 1-Columnar epithelium. 2-Stratified squamous lining of lower end of oesophagus. 3-Gastric pit. 4-Cardiac gland. 5-Oesophageal gland. 6-Muscularis mucosae. 7-Submucosa. 8-Circular muscle. 9-Longitudinal muscle.

Stomach, Cardiac End

The cardiac end of the stomach is lined by columnar cells (1). The epithelium is sharply demarcated from the stratified squamous epithelium lining the lower end of the oesophagus (2).

The mucosa of the stomach shows a number of shallow depressions called gastric pits (3) deep to which there are cardiac glands (4).

Some oesophageal (mucous) glands (5) are seen in the submucosa (7). A muscularis mucosae (6), and circular (8) and longitudinal (9) coats of muscle are present.

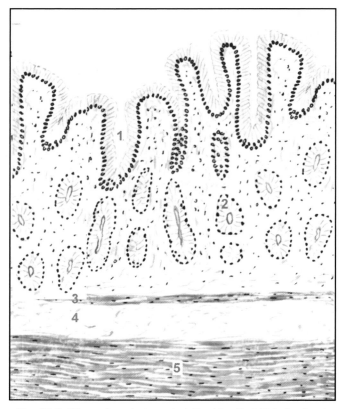

Fig. 13.6. Stomach, pyloric part. 1-Gastric pit. 2-Pyloric gland. 3-Muscularis mucosae. 4-Submucosa. 5. Circular muscle.

The Pyloric Glands

In the pyloric region of the stomach the gastric pits are deep and occupy two thirds of the depth of the mucosa. The pyloric glands that open into these pits are short and occupy the deeper one third of the mucosa. They are simple or branched tubular glands that are coiled. The glands are lined by mucous secreting cells. Occasional oxyntic and argentaffin cells may be present. Some pyloric glands may pass through the muscularis mucosae to enter the submucosa. In addition to other substances, pyloric glands secrete the hormone gastrin.

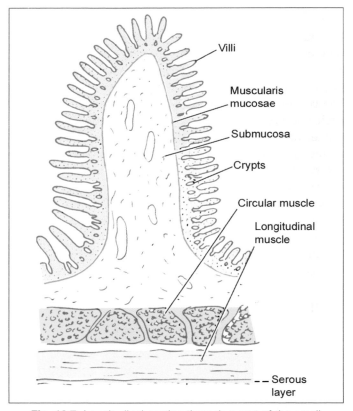

Fig. 13.7. Longitudinal section through a part of the small intestine seen at a very low magnification to show a mucosal fold.

Small Intestine: Basic Structure

The mucous membrane of the small intestine shows distinctive features. These are (a) circular folds, (b) villi and (c) crypts.

Circular Folds

The circular folds are also called the **valves of Kerkring**. Each fold is made up of all layers of the mucosa (lining epithelium, lamina propria and muscularis mucosae). The submucosa also extends into the folds. The folds are large and readily seen with the naked eye. They are absent in the first one or two inches of the duodenum. They are prominent in the rest of the duodenum, and in the whole of the jejunum. The folds gradually become fewer and less marked in the ileum. The terminal parts of the ileum have no such folds.

Apart from adding considerably to the surface area of the mucous membrane, the circular folds tend to slow down the passage of contents through the small intestine thus facilitating absorption.

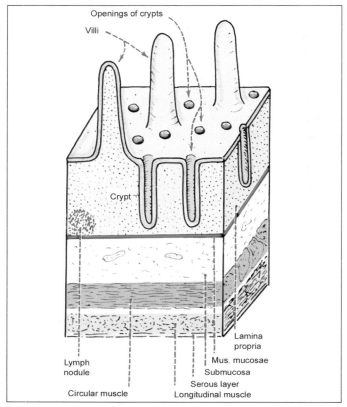

Fig. 13.8. Scheme to show the basic structure of the small intestine.

Small Intestine: The Villi

The villi are, typically, finger like projections consisting of a core of reticular tissue covered by a surface epithelium (described below). The connective tissue core contains numerous blood capillaries forming a plexus. The endothelium lining the capillaries is fenestrated thus allowing rapid absorption of nutrients into the blood. Each villus contains a central lymphatic vessel called a *lacteal*. Distally, the lacteal ends blindly near the tip of the villus; and proximally it ends in a plexus of lymphatic vessels present in the lamina propria. Occasionally, the lacteal may be double. Some muscle fibres derived from the muscularis mucosae extend into the villus core.

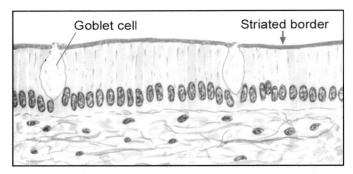

Fig. 13.9. Columnar epithelium lining the small intestine.
Note the striated border and some goblet cells.

Small Intestine: The Epithelial Lining

The epithelium covering the villi, and areas of the mucosal surface intervening between them, consists predominantly of columnar cells that are specialized for absorption. These are called **enterocytes**. Scattered amongst the columnar cells there are mucous secreting goblet cells. The cells lining the crypts (intestinal glands) are predominantly undifferentiated. These cells multiply to give rise to absorptive columnar cells and to goblet cells. Near the bases of the crypts there are **Paneth cells** that secrete enzymes (Page 143). Endocrine cells (bearing membrane bound granules filled with various neuroactive peptides) are also present (Page 144).

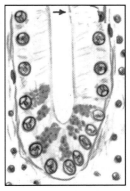

Fig. 13.10. Paneth cell.

Zymogen Cells (Paneth Cells)

These cells are found only in the deeper parts of intestinal crypts. They contain prominent eosinophilic secretory granules. They may produce various enzymes.

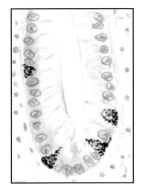

Fig. 13.11. Argentaffin cell.

Endocrine Cells

As the granules in them stain with silver salts these cells are also argentaffin cells. They are called ***enterochromaffin cells***.

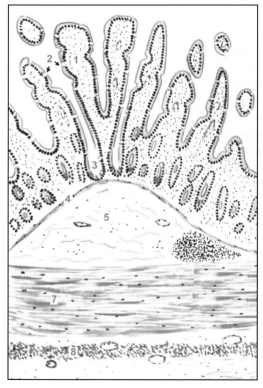

Fig. 13.12. Jejunum. 1-Villus. 2-Goblet cells. 3-Crypt. 4- Muscularis mucosae. 5-Submucosa. 6-Note the solitary lymphatic nodule seen towards the right side. 7-Circular muscle. 8-Longitudinal muscle.

Jejunum

In this figure we see features of the typical structure of the small intestine. The mucosa shows numerous finger like projections or villi (1). Each villus has a covering of columnar epithelium that covers a core of delicate connective tissue. Some goblet cells (2) are also seen. Numerous tubular depressions, or crypts (3) dip into the lamina propria. These crypts are also lined by columnar cells. The mucosa is separated from the submucosa (5) by the muscularis mucosae (4). A solitary lymph nodule (6) is present in the submucosa. The intestine is surrounded by circular (7) and longitudinal (8) layers of smooth muscle.

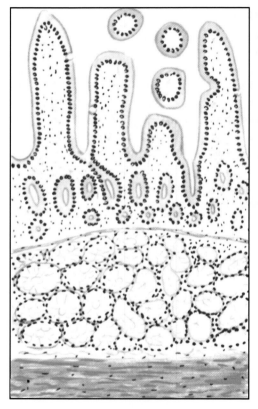

Fig. 13.13. Duodenum. Note that the submucosa is packed with mucous secreting glands (of Brunner).

Duodenum

The general structure of the duodenum is the same as that described for the jejunum, except that the submucosa is packed with mucous secreting glands of Brunner. Note that the intestinal crypts lie 'above' the muscularis mucosae while the glands of Brunner lie 'below' it. The presence of the glands of Brunner is a distinctive feature of the duodenum.

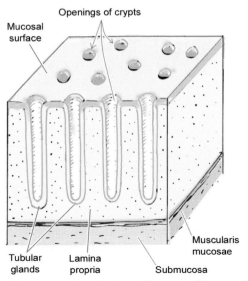

Fig. 13.14. Scheme to show the basic features of the structure of the mucous membrane of the large intestine. Also see page 148

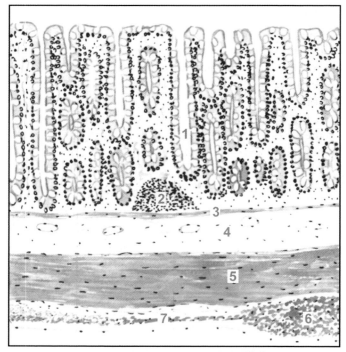

Fig. 13.15. Section through a part of the large intestine. 1-Crypt. 2-Lymphatic nodule. 3-Muscularis mucosae. 4-Submucosa. 5-Muscle coat. 6-Taenia coli. 7-Longitudinal muscle.

Large Intestine

The mucosa shows numerous tubular glands or crypts (1). The surface of the mucosa, and the crypts, are lined by columnar cells amongst which there are numerous goblet cells. A section of the large intestine is easily distinguished from that of the small intestine because of the absence of villi; and from the stomach because of the presence of goblet cells (which are absent in the stomach). Crypts of the large intestine do not show Paneth cells, but argentaffin cells are present. A lymphatic nodule (2) is seen in the lamina propria. The muscularis mucosae (3), submucosa (4) and circular muscle coat (5) are similar to those in the small intestine. However, the longitudinal muscle coat is gathered into three thick bands called taenia coli, one of which is seen at '6'. The longitudinal muscle is thin in the intervals between the taenia (7).

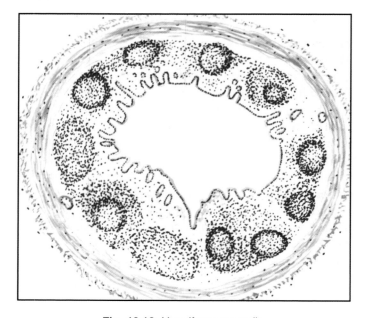

Fig. 13.16. Vermiform appendix.
Note the lymphatic nodules filling the submucosa almost completely.

The Vermiform Appendix

The structure of the vermiform appendix resembles that of the colon (described above) with the following differences (Fig. 13.16).

1. The appendix is the narrowest part of the gut.

2. The crypts are poorly formed.

3. The longitudinal muscle coat is complete and equally thick all round. Taenia coli are not present.

4. The submucosa contains abundant lymphoid tissue that may completely fill the submucosa. The lymphoid tissue is not present at birth. It gradually increases and is best seen in children about 10 years old. Subsequently, there is progressive reduction in quantity of lymphoid tissue.

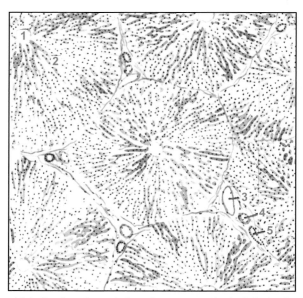

Fig. 14.1. Section through liver (low power view). 1-Central vein. 2-Liver cells arranged as radiating cords or plates that form hexagonal lobules. 3-Branch of portal vein. 4- Branch of hepatic artery. 5-Interlobular duct. 3, 4 and 5 form a portal triad.

Liver

In Figure 14.1 we see a low power view. The substance of the liver is made up of liver cells (hepatocytes) arranged in the form of hexagonal areas called hepatic lobules. The lobules are partially separated by connective tissue. Each lobule has a central vein (1) from which numerous sinusoids (seen as empty spaces) pass radially. The spaces between the sinusoids are occupied by plates of liver cells: the plates look like cords when seen in section (2), Along the periphery of the lobules there are angular intervals filled by connective tissue. Each such area contains a branch of the portal vein (3), a branch of the hepatic artery (4), and an interlobular bile duct (5). These three constitute a portal triad.

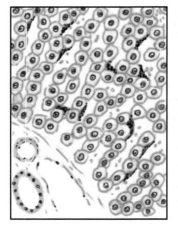 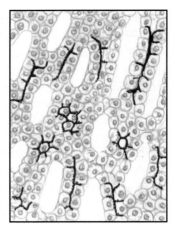

Fig. 14.2   Fig. 14.3

These are high power views of the liver. In **Figure 14.2** note cords of cells separated by sinusoids. Phagocytic cells (of Kupffer) (containing dark injested material) are seen scattered along the walls of sinusoids. In **Figure 14.3** note the bile capillaries (black) intervening between liver cells.

In Figures 14.2 and 14.3 we see parts of the liver at higher magnification. Polygonal liver cells arranged in a radial manner, separated by sinusoids, are seen. In Figure 14.2 the tissue has been specially prepared to show phagocytic cells (of Kupffer) (arrows) in the walls of sinusoids. Particles of black ink injected into the circulation of the living animal have been taken up by these cells.In Figure 14.3 the tissue has been prepared to demonstrate bile capillaries (arrows) present in the intervals between liver cells.

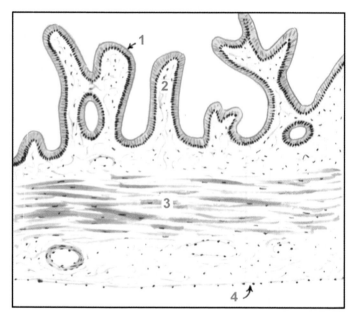

Fig. 14.4. Gallbladder. 1- Mucous membrane lined by columnar epithelium. 2-Mucosal fold. 3-Muscle coat. 4-Serous layer (peritoneum) lined by flattened mesothelium.

Gallbladder

The mucous membrane is lined by tall columnar cells (1). The mucosa is highly folded and some of the folds (2) might look like villi. Because of this beginners might confuse sections of the gallbladder with those of the small intestine. Distinction is easy if it is remembered that in the gallbladder there are no goblet cells, and no muscularis mucosae. The muscle coat (3) is poorly developed there being numerous connective tissue fibres amongst the muscle fibres. A serous covering (4) lined by flattened mesothelium is seen.

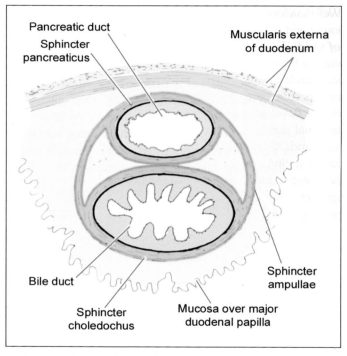

Fig. 14.5. Section through the major duodenal papilla to show the components of the sphincter of Oddi.

Well developed smooth muscle is present in the region of the lower end of the bile duct. This muscle forms the ***sphincter of Oddi***. From a functional point of view this sphincter consists of three separate parts. The ***sphincter choledochus*** surrounds the lower end of the bile duct. It is always present, and its contraction is responsible for filling of the gallbladder. A less developed ***sphincter pancreaticus*** surrounds the terminal part of the main pancreatic duct. A third sphincter surrounds the hepato-pancreatic duct (or ampulla) and often forms a ring round the lower ends of both the bile and pancreatic ducts. This is the ***sphincter ampullae***. The sphincter ampullae and the sphincter pancreaticus are often missing.

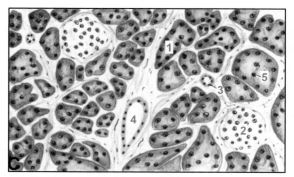

Fig. 14.6. Pancreas. 1-Serous acini. 2-Pancreatic islet. 3-Intralobular duct. 4-Interlobular duct.

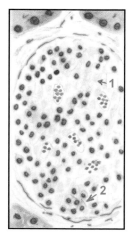

Fig. 14.7. Pancreatic islet. 1-Alpha cells. 2-Beta cells. 3-Capillary.

Pancreas

This is a compound tubulo-alveolar gland made up of serous acini (1) and, therefore, resembling the parotid gland. The two are, however, easily distinguished because of the presence (in the pancreas) of groups of cells that form the pancreatic islets (2): these islets are endocrine in function. Intralobular ducts (3) are few. n interlobular duct is shown at 4. The cells forming the acini of the pancreas are highly basophilic. The lumen of the acinus is seldom seen. The central parts of acini are occupied by centroacinar cells (5). In Figure 14.7 we see a high power view of a pancreatic islet. The preparation has been specially stained to differentiate between alpha cells (1) that are stained pink, and beta cells (2) that are stained bluish. A number of capillaries (3) are seen.

CHAPTER FIFTEEN

The Urinary Organs

Kidney (Low Power View)

In Figure 15.1 we see a section through part of a kidney at low magnification. The kidney is covered by a capsule (1). Deep to the capsule there is the cortex (occupying the upper 4/5 of the figure). In the cortex we see circular structures called renal corpuscles (2) surrounding which there are tubules cut in various shapes. The dark pink stained tubules are parts of the proximal convoluted tubules (3): their lumen is small and indistinct. Lighter staining tubules, each with a distinct lumen, are the distal convoluted tubules (4). An artery is seen at '5', and a vein at '6'. The very light staining, elongated, parallel running tubules seen in the medulla (8) are collecting ducts. Some of them extend into the cortex (7) forming a medullary ray.

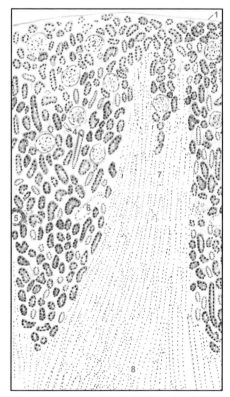

Fig. 15.1. Kidney (low power view). 1-Capsule, 2-Renal corpuscle. 3-Proximal convoluted tubule. 4-Distal convoluted tubule. 5-Artery. 6-Vein. 7-Medullary ray. 8-Collecting duct.

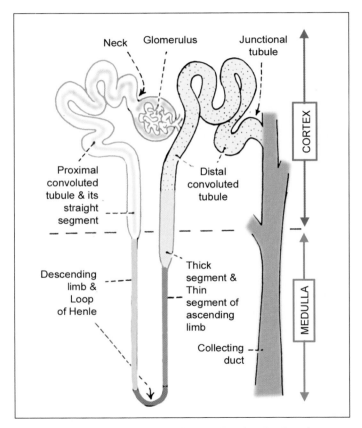

Fig. 15.2. Parts of a nephron. A collecting duct is also shown.

Parts of the Nephron

The nephron consists of a **renal corpuscle** (or **Malpighian corpuscle**), and a long complicated **renal tubule**. The renal corpuscle is a rounded structure consisting of (a) a rounded tuft of blood capillaries called the **glomerulus**; and (b) a cup-like, double layered covering for the glomerulus called the **glomerular capsule** (or **Bowman's capsule**). The glomerular capsule represents the cup-shaped blind beginning of the renal tubule. Between the two layers of the capsule there is a **urinary space** that is continuous with the lumen of the renal tubule.

The renal tubule is divisible into several parts that are shown in Figure 15.2. Starting from the glomerular capsule there are: (**a**) the **proximal convoluted tubule**; (**b**) the **loop of Henle** consisting of a **descending limb**, a **loop**, and an **ascending limb**; and (**c**) the **distal convoluted tubule**, which ends by joining a collecting tubule.

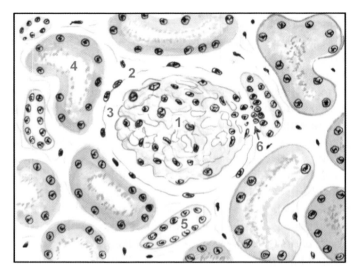

Fig. 15.3. Renal cortex (high power view). 1-Glomerulus. 2-Glomerular capsule. 3-Urinary space. 4-Proximal convoluted tubule. 5-Distal convoluted tubule. 6-Macula densa.

Renal Cortex (High Power View)

In this figure we see a high power view of the cortex. Note the large renal corpuscle consisting of a tuft of capillaries that form a rounded glomerulus (1), and an outer wall, the glomerular capsule (2). Note the urinary space (3) between the glomerulus and the capsule. Proximal convoluted tubules (4) are dark staining. They are lined by cuboidal cells with a prominent brush border. Distal convoluted tubules (5) are lighter staining. The cuboidal cells lining them do not have a brush border. Their lumen is distinct. At '6' we see a distal convoluted tubule closely related to the renal corpuscle. The nuclei in part of its wall are closely packed to form a structure called the macula densa: the macula is part of an important region called the juxtaglomerular apparatus. For a high power view of the renal medulla see Figure 15.4.

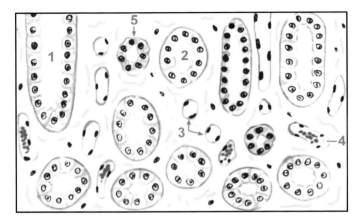

Fig. 15.4. Renal medulla (high power view). 1, 2-Collecting duct (L.S & T.S). 3, 5-Loop of Henle (thin and thick segments). 4-Capillary.

Renal Medulla (High Power View)

This is a high power view of a part of the medulla. Note the following:

(a) A number of collecting ducts cut longitudinally (1) or transversely (2) are seen. They are lined by a cuboidal epithelium, the cells of which stain lightly. Cell boundaries are usually distinct. The lumen of the tubule is also distinct.

(b) Sections of the thin segment of the loop of Henle are seen at '3': they are lined by flattened cells, the walls being very similar in appearance to those of blood capillaries (4).

(c) Sections through the thick segments of loops of Henle are seen at '5': they are lined by cuboidal epithelium.

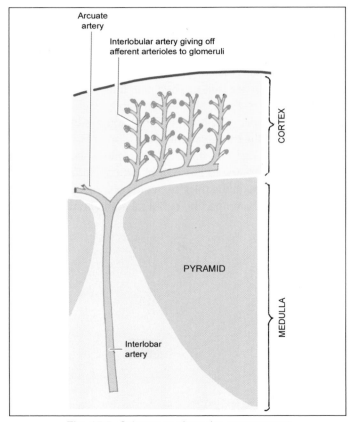

Fig. 15.5. Scheme to show the arrangement
of arteries within the kidney.

At the hilum of the kidney each renal artery divides into a number of *lobar arteries* (one for each pyramid). Each lobar artery divides into two (or more) *interlobar arteries* that enter the tissue of the renal columns and run towards the surface of the kidney. Reaching the level of the bases of the pyramids, the interlobar arteries divide into *arcuate arteries*. The arcuate arteries run at right angles to the parent interlobar arteries.

They lie parallel to the renal surface at the junction of the pyramid and the cortex. They give off a series of *interlobular arteries* that run through the cortex at right angles to the renal surface to end in a subcapsular plexus. Each interlobular artery gives off a series of arterioles that enter glomeruli as *afferent arterioles*.

Blood from these arterioles circulates through gomerular capillaries that join to form *efferent arterioles* that emerge from glomeruli.

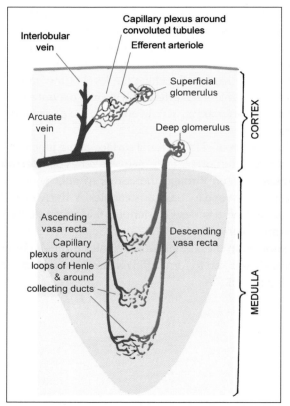

Fig. 15.6. Scheme to show behaviour of efferent arterioles of glomeruli in the superficial and deeper parts of the renal cortex.

The behaviour of efferent arterioles leaving the glomeruli differs in the case of glomeruli located more superficially in the cortex, and those lying near the pyramids. Efferent arterioles arising from the majority of glomeruli (superficial) divide into capillaries that surround the proximal and distal convoluted tubules. These capillaries drain into **interlobular veins**, and through them into **arcuate veins** and **interlobar veins**. Efferent arterioles arising from glomeruli nearer the medulla (**juxtamedullary glomeruli**) divide into 12 to 25 straight vessels that descend into the medulla. These are the **descending vasa recta**. Side branches arising from the vasa recta join a capillary plexus that surrounds the descending and ascending limbs of the loop of Henle (and also the collecting tubules). The capillary plexus consists predominantly of vessels running longitudinally along the tubules. It is drained by **ascending vasa recta** that run upwards parallel to the descending vasa recta to reach the cortex. Here they drain into interlobular or arcuate veins.

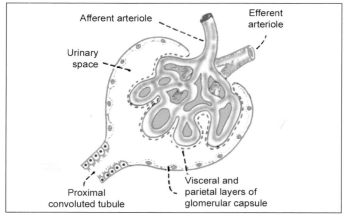

Fig. 15.7. Scheme to show the basic structure
of a renal corpuscle.

Renal Corpuscle

The glomerulus is a rounded tuft of anastomosing capillaries. Blood enters the tuft through an afferent arteriole and leaves it through an efferent arteriole.

The afferent and efferent arterioles lie close together at a point that is referred to as the ***vascular pole*** of the renal corpuscle. The glomerular capsule is a double-layered cup, the two layers of which are separated by the urinary space. The outer layer is lined by squamous cells. With the light microscope the inner wall also appears to be lined by squamous cells, but the EM shows that these cells, called

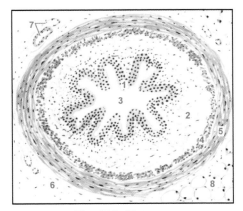

Fig. 15.8. Ureter.

podocytes, have a highly specialized structure. The urinary space becomes continuous with the lumen of the renal tubule at the **urinary pole** of the renal corpuscle. This pole lies diametrically opposite the vascular pole.

Ureter

The mucous membrane is lined by transitional epithelium (1)which rests on a layer of connective tissue (2). The mucosa shows folds that give the lumen a star shaped appearance (3). The muscle coat has an inner layer of longitudinal fibres (4) and an outer layer of circular fibres (5). Note that this arrangement is the reverse of that in the gut. The muscle coat is surrounded by connective tissue (6) in which blood vessels (7) and fat cells (8) are present.

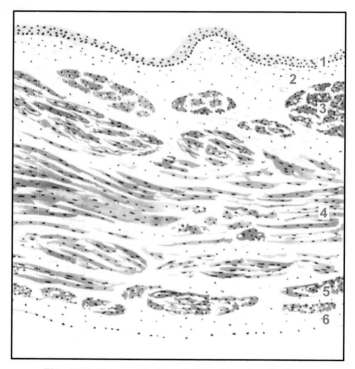

Fig. 15.9. Urinary bladder. 1-Transitional epithelium.
2-Connective tissue. 3, 4, 5-Muscle layers.

Urinary Bladder

The wall of the urinary bladder consists of an outer serous layer, a thick coat of smooth muscle, and a mucous membrane. The mucous membrane is lined by transitional epithelium. The epithelium rests on a layer of loose fibrous tissue. There is no muscularis mucosae.

When the bladder is distended (with urine) the lining epithelium becomes thinner.

In the empty bladder the mucous membrane is thrown into numerous folds (or rugae) that disappear when the bladder is distended. Some mucous glands may be present in the mucosa specially near the internal urethral orifice.

The muscle layer is thick. The smooth muscle in it forms a meshwork. Internally and externally the fibres tend to be longitudinal. In between them there is a thicker layer of circular (or oblique) fibres. Contraction of this muscle coat is responsible for emptying of the bladder.

CHAPTER SIXTEEN

The Male Reproductive Organs

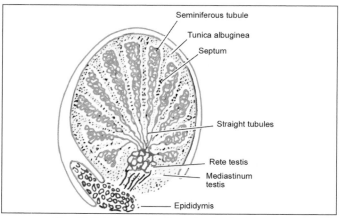

Fig. 16.1. Scheme to show the basic structure of the testis.

Testis

Each testis is an oval structure about 4 cm long. The outermost layer of the organ is formed by a dense fibrous membrane called the **tunica albuginea**. In the posterior part of the testis the connective tissue of the tunica albuginea expands into a thick mass that projects into the substance of the testis.

This projection is called the ***mediastinum testis***. Numerous septa pass from the mediastinum testis to the tunica albuginea, and divide the substance of the testis into a large number of lobules. Each obule is roughly conical, the apex of the cone being directed towards the mediastinum testis. Each lobule contains one or more highly convoluted ***seminiferous tubules***.

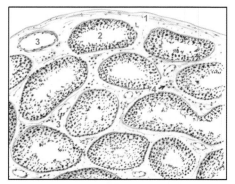

Fig. 16.2. Testis, low power view. 1-Tunica albuginea. 2-Seminiferous tubule. 3-Blood vessel. 4-Interstitial cells.

In Figure 16.2 we see a low power view. The testis has an outer fibrous layer, the tunica albuginea (1) deep to which are seen a number of seminiferous tubules (2) cut in various directions.

The tubules are separated by connective tissue, containing blood vessels (3) and groups of interstitial cells (4). Each seminiferous tubule is lined by several layers of cells.

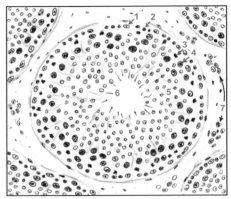

Fig. 16.3. Testis, high power view. 1-Sustentacular cells. 2-Spermatogonia. 3-Dividing spermatogonia. 4-Spermatocyte. 5-Spermatid. 6-Spermatozoa. 7-Interstitial cells.

Figure 16.3 shows details of cells lining a seminiferous tubule seen at a high magnification. Note that the cell boundaries are indistinct, and nuclei are prominent.

The outermost row of nuclei belongs to sustentacular cells (1) and to spermatogonia (2), some of which are undergoing mitosis (3: note very dense nucleus of irregular shape). Passing inwards towards the centre of the tubule we have large darkly staining nuclei of spermatocytes (4), and many smaller nuclei of spermatids (5). Towards the centre of the tubule a number of developing spermatozoa are seen (6). Note groups of interstitial cells (7) in the connective tissue between the seminiferous tubules.

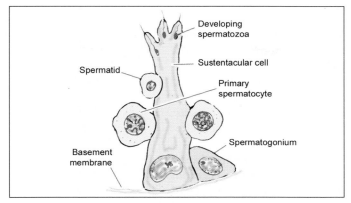

Fig. 16.4. Scheme to show a sustentacular cell and some related germ cells.

Sustentacular Cells or Cells of Sertoli

These are tall, slender cells having an irregularly pyramidal or columnar shape. The nucleus lies near the base of the cell. It is light staining and is of irregular shape. There is a prominent nucleolus. The base of each sustentacular cell rests on the basement membrane, spermatogonia being interposed amongst the sustentacular cells. The apex of the sustentacular cell reaches the lumen of the seminiferous tubule. Numerous spermatids, at various stages of differentiation into spermatozoa, appear to be embedded in the apical part of the cytoplasm. Nearer the basement membrane spermatocytes and spermatogonia indent the sustentacular cell cytoplasm.

Spermatozoon

The spermatozoon has a **head**, a **neck**, a **middle piece** and a **principal piece** or **tail**. The head is covered by a cap called the **acrosomic cap**, **anterior nuclear cap**, or **galea capitis**.

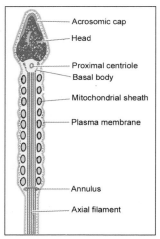

The neck of the spermatozoon is narrow. It contains a funnel-shaped **basal body** and a spherical **centriole**. An **axial filament** (or **axoneme**) begins just behind this centriole. It passes through the middle piece and extends into the tail. At the point where the middle piece joins the tail, this axial filament

Fig. 16.5. Structure of a spermatozoon as seen by EM.

passes through a ring-like **annulus**. That part of the axial filament that lies in the middle piece is surrounded by a **spiral sheath** made up of mitochondria.

The **head** of the human spermatozoon is flattened from before backwards so that it is oval when seen from the front, but appears to be pointed (somewhat like a spear-head) when seen from one side, or in section. It consists of chromatin (mostly DNA) that is extremely condensed and, therefore, appears to have a homogeneous structure even when examined by EM. This condensation makes it highly resistant to various physical stresses.

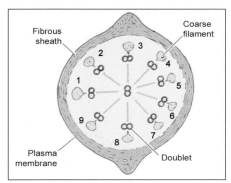

Fig. 16.6. Transverse section across the tail of a spermatozoon to show the arrangement of fibrils.

The chief structure to be seen in the neck is the ***basal body***. It is also called the ***connecting piece*** because it helps to establish an intimate union between the head and the remainder of the spermatozoon. The basal body is made up of nine segmented rod-like structures each of which is continuous distally with one coarse fibre of the axial filament (see below). On its proximal side (i.e. towards the head of the spermatozoon) the basal body has a convex ***articular surface*** that fits into a depression (called the ***implantation fossa***) present in the head.

The ***axial filament***, that passes through the middle piece and most of the tail, is really composed of several fibrils arranged as illustrated in Figure 16.6. There is a pair of central fibrils, surrounded by nine pairs (or ***doublets***) arranged in a circle around the central pair. (This arrangement of one central pair of fibrils surrounded by nine doublets is similar to that seen in cilia).

In addition to these doublets there are nine coarser petal-shaped fibrils of unequal size, one such fibril lying just outside each doublet.

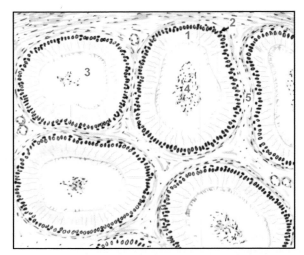

Fig. 16.7. Epidydimis. 1-Lining of tall columnar cells. 2-Basal cell.
3-Stereocilia. 4-Clump of spermatozoa.

Epididymis

The section passes through the body of the epididymis which
consists of a long convoluted duct which is cut up several
times.

The duct is lined by pseudostratified columnar epithelium
in which there are tall columnar cells (1) and shorter basal
cells (2) that do not reach the lumen. The columnar cells
bear stereocilia (3) that are non-motile.

Clumps of spermatozoa (4) are present in the lumen. Note
the smooth muscle (5) in the wall of the duct.

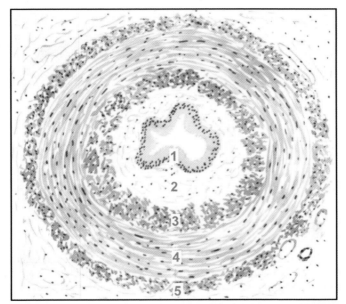

Fig. 16.8. Ductus deferens. 1-Pseudostratified columnar epithelium. 2-Lamina propria. 3, 4, 5-Muscle layers (inner longitudinal, middle circular, outer longitudinal).

Ductus Deferens

The mucous membrane is lined by pseudostratified columnar epithelium (1) which rests on a lamina propria (2). The muscle coat is very thick. Three layers, inner longitudinal (3), middle circular (4) and outer longitudinal (5) are seen.

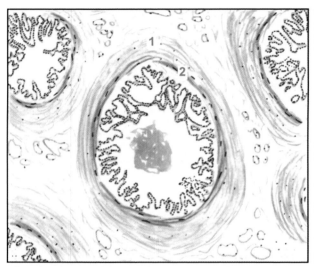

Fig. 16.9. Seminal vesicle (low power). It is made up of a convoluted tubule that is cut up several times. 1-Connective tissue. 2-Smooth muscle.

Seminal Vesicle

It is made up of a convoluted tubule which is cut up several times in any section. The tube has an outer covering of connective tissue (1), a thin layer of smooth muscle (2) and an inner mucosa. The mucosal lining is thrown into numerous folds that branch and anastomose to form a network. The lining epithelium is simple columnar or pseudostratified.

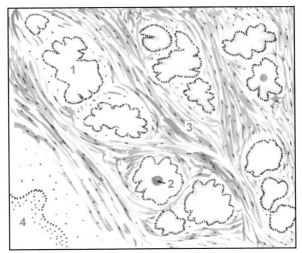

Fig. 16.10. Prostate (low power view). 1-Follicle of irregular shape. 2-Amyloid body. 3-Fibromuscular tissue. 4-Prostatic urethra lined by transitional epithelium.

Prostate

The prostate consists of glandular tissue embedded in prominent fibro-muscular tissue. The glandular tissue is in the form of follicles of irregular shape (1) that are lined by columnar epithelium. The lumen may contain amyloid bodies (2). The follicles are separated by broad bands of fibromuscular tissue (3): This tissue is a characteristic feature of the prostate. The prostate is traversed by the prostatic urethra (4) which is lined by transitional epithelium.

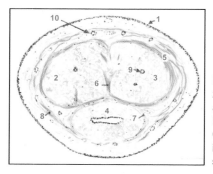

Fig. 16.11. Penis. 1-Skin. 2, 3, 5-Corpora cavernosa and sheaths for them. 6-Median septum. 4,7-Corpus spongiosum and its sheath. 8-Common sheath. 10-Dorsal artery.

Penis

This figure shows a transverse section through the body of the penis seen at very low magnification.

The penis has an outer covering of skin (1). The substance of the organ is made up of three masses of erectile tissue. Two masses, placed side by side, towards the dorsum, are the right and left corpora cavernosa (2,3). One mass lying in the midline, ventral to the corpora cavernosa is the corpus spongiosum (4). This is traversed by the penile urethra. Each corpus cavernosum is surrounded by a thick fibrous sheath (5) which also forms a median septum (6). The corpus spongiosum has a thinner sheath (7). There is an additional sheath (8) common to all three masses of erectile tissue. Note the artery in the centre of each corpus cavernosum (9), the two dorsal arteries (10), and numerous other vessels.

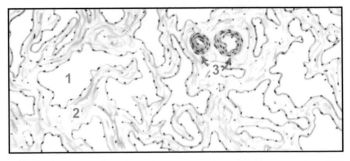

Fig. 16.12. Erectile tissue (from part of penis). 1-space lined by endothelium. 2-Connective tissue. 3-Artery with thick muscular wall.

Penis: Erectile Tissue

This figure is a high power view of erectile tissue (present in the penis). This tissue consists of numerous spaces (1) that are lined by endothelium. The spaces are separated by a network of connective tissue (2). Two arteries (3) with thick muscular walls are seen.

CHAPTER SEVENTEEN
The Female
Reproductive Organs

Ovary (Low Power View)

The surface is covered by a cuboidal epithelium (1). Deep to the epithelium there is a layer of connective tissue that constitutes the tunica albuginea (2). The substance of the ovary shows an outer cortex in which follicles of various sizes are present (3,4); and an inner medulla consisting of connective tissue containing blood vessels (16). Just deep to the tunica albuginea we see many primordial follicles (5) each of which contains a developing ovum surrounded by flattened follicular cells. Somewhat more developed ovarian follicles are seen at '6'. A large follicle is seen at '7'. It has a follicular cavity (7) surrounded by several layers of follicular cells (8). On one side there is a developing ovum (9). The cells surrounding the ovum constitute the cumulus oophoricus (10). The follicle is surrounded by a capsule (11) for it. The follicle is surrounded by a stroma (12). At '13' we have another follicle in which an ovum is not seen as the section does not pass through the plane in which the ovum lies. At '14' we see a structure called the corpus luteum. At '15' we see two rounded masses of fibrous tissue that represent remnants of degenerated or atretic follicles.

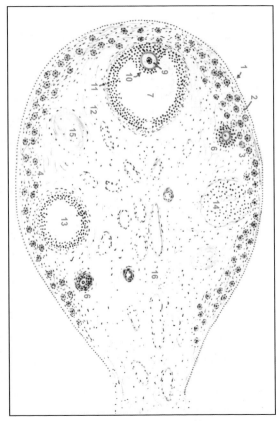

Fig. 17.1. Ovary, panoramic view.

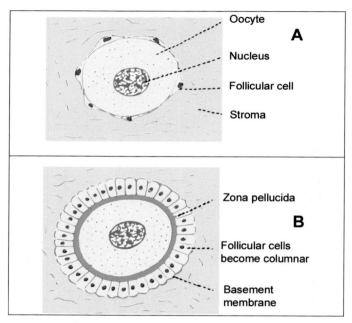

Fig. 17.2. Diagrammatic presentation of:
A. Primordial follicle. B. Primary follicle.

Ovarian follicles (or *Graafian follicles*) are derived from stromal cells that surround developing ova as follows.

1. Some cells of the stroma become flattened and surround an oocyte (Fig. 17.2A). These stromal cells are now called *follicular cells*.

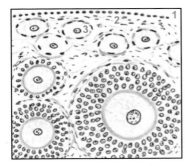

Fig. 17.3. Section of ovary (high power) showing early stages in formation of follicles. 1-Germinal epithelium. 2-Tunica albuginea. 3-Primordial follicle. One primary follicle and two secondary follicles are also seen.

The ovum and the flat surrounding cells form a ***primordial follicle***. Numerous primordial follicles are present in the ovary at birth. They undergo further development only at puberty.

2. The first indication that a primordial follicle is beginning to undergo further development is that the flattened follicular cells become columnar (Fig. 17.2B). Follicles at this stage of development are called ***primary follicles***.

3. A homogeneous membrane, the ***zona pellucida***, appears between the follicular cells and the oocyte (Fig.17.2B). With the appearance of the zona pellucida the follicle is now referred to as a ***multilaminar primary follicle***

4. The follicular cells proliferate to form several layers of cells that constitute the ***membrana granulosa***. The cells are now called ***granulosa cells***. This is a ***secondary follicle***.

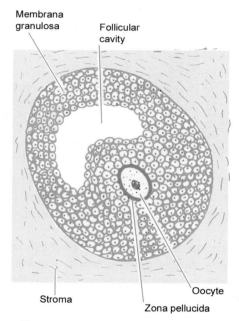

Membrana granulosa

Follicular cavity

Oocyte

Stroma

Zona pellucida

Fig. 17.4. Developing ovarian follicle after establishment of a follicular cavity.

5. So far the granulosa cells are in the form of a compact mass. However, the cells to one side of the ovum soon partially separate from one another so that a *follicular cavity* (or *antrum folliculi*) appears between them. It is with the appearance of this cavity that a true follicle (= small sac) can

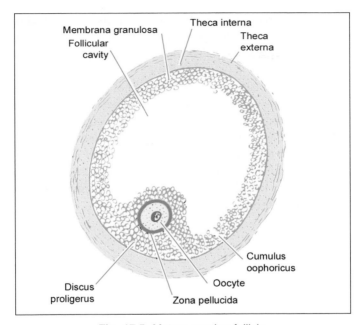

Fig. 17.5. Mature ovarian follicle.

be said to have been formed. The follicular cavity is filled by a fluid, the ***liquor folliculi*** (Fig. 17.4).

6. The follicular cavity rapidly increases in size. As a result, the wall of the follicle (formed by the granulosa cells) becomes relatively thin (Fig. 17.5). The oocyte now lies eccentrically in the follicle surrounded by some granulosa cells that are given the name of **cumulus oophoricus** (or **cumulus oophorus**, or **cumulus ovaricus**). The granulosa cells that attach the oocyte to the wall of the follicle constitute the **discus proligerus**.

7. As the follicle expands the stromal cells surrounding the membrana granulosa become condensed to form a covering called the **theca interna** (theca = cover). The cells of the theca interna later secrete a hormone called **oestrogen**, and they are then called the cells of the **thecal gland**.

8. Outside the theca interna some fibrous tissue becomes condensed to form another covering for the follicle. This is the **theca externa**.

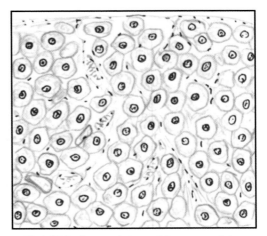

Fig. 17.6. Corpus luteum (diagrammatic).
Note the large hexagonal cells filled with yellow granules.

Corpus Luteum

The corpus luteum is an important structure. It secretes a hormone, ***progesterone***. The corpus luteum is derived from the ovarian follicle, after the latter has ruptured to shed the ovum, as follows.

(a) When the follicle ruptures its wall collapses and becomes folded. Sudden reduction in pressure caused by rupture of the follicle results in bleeding into the follicle. The follicle filled with blood is called the ***corpus haemorrhagicum***.

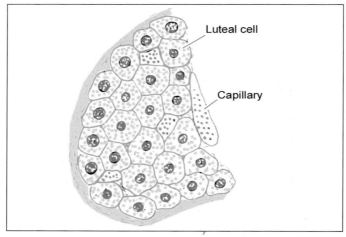

Fig. 17.7. Corpus luteum as seen in a section after haemataoxylin and eosin staining (high power view). Note large polyhedral cells and capillaries present amongst them.

(**b**) At this stage, the follicular cells are small and rounded. They now enlarge rapidly. As they increase in size their walls press against those of neighbouring cells so that the cells acquire a polyhedral shape (Fig. 17.6). Their cytoplasm becomes filled with a yellow pigment called **lutein**. They are now called **luteal cells**. The presence of this yellow pigment gives the structure a yellow colour, and that is why it is called the corpus luteum (= yellow body).

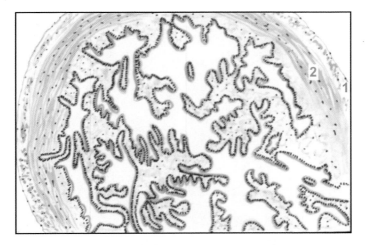

Fig. 17.8. Uterine tube. 1,2-Muscle layer (longitudinal and circular). Mucous membrane shows branching folds covered by ciliated columnar epithelium.

Uterine Tube

The uterine tube has a muscular wall with an outer longitudinal (1) and inner circular (2) layer. The mucous membrane shows numerous branching folds which almost fill the lumen of the tube. The mucosa is lined by ciliated columnar epithelium.

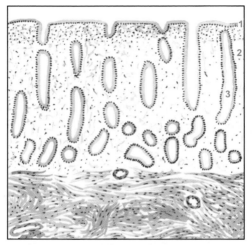

Fig. 17.9. Uterus (Proliferative phase). 1-Lining of columnar epithelium. 2-Stroma. 3-Uterine gland. Also observe the muscular coat.

Uterus

The wall of the uterus consists of a mucous membrane (called the endometrium) and a very thick layer of muscle (the myometrium). Only a very small part of the myometrium is included in these figures.

The endometrium has a lining of columnar epithelium (1) that rests on a stroma of connective tissue (2). Numerous tubular uterine glands (3) dip into the stroma.

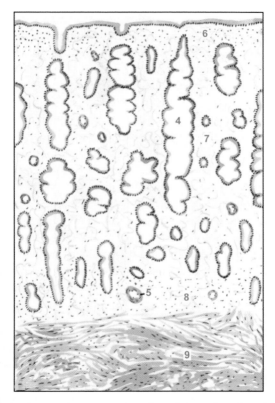

Fig. 17.10. Uterus (secretory phase). 4-Enlarged uterine gland. 5-Artery. 6-Stratum compactum. 7-Stratum spongiosum. 8-Stratum basale. 9-Muscle layer.

The appearance of the endometrium varies considerably depending upon the phase of the menstrual cycle.

In Figure 17.9 the endometrium is shown in the proliferative phase; while in Figure 17.10 it is shown in the secretory phase. In the proliferative phase the endometrium is relatively thin, and the glands in it are straight (3). In the secretory phase the thickness of the endometrium is much increased. The uterine glands elongate, become dilated, and tortuous as a result of which they have saw-toothed margins in sections (4). Blood vessels become more conspicuous (5). The stroma becomes divisible into three parts: there is a superficial stratum compactum (6) in which the cells are closely packed, a middle stratum spongiosum (7) which is relatively loose, and a stratum basale (8) in which the cells are again densely packed (as indicated by density of nuclei).

The myometrium is described as having various layers, but these are difficult to make out as the fibres run in various directions (9).

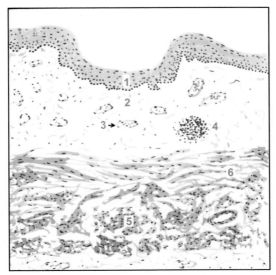

Fig. 17.11. Vagina. 1-Lining of stratified squamous epithelium. 2-Connective tissue. 3-Blood vessels. 4-Lymphoid follicle. 5,6-Muscle coat (longitudinal and circular).

Vagina

The vagina has a mucosa which is lined by stratified squamous epithelium (non-keratinized) (1) that rests on connective tissue (2) in which there are many blood vessels (3). Lymphoid follicles (4) are also present. There are no glands in the mucosa. The muscle coat has an outer layer of longitudinal fibres (5) and a thin inner layer of circular fibres (6).

CHAPTER EIGHTEEN

The Endocrine System

Hypophysis Cerebri

In Figure 18.1 we see the pars anterior of the hypophysis cerebri. This part consists of groups or cords of cells with numerous sinusoids between them. The cells are of three types. The pink staining cells (1) are alpha cells or acidophils. The cells with bluish cytoplasm (2) are beta cells or basophils. Cells in which the cytoplasm is not conspicuous, and the nuclei are closely packed, are chromophobe cells.

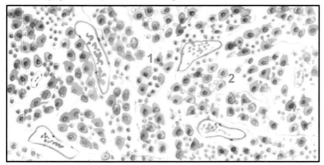

Fig. 18.1. Hypophysis cerebri. Pars anterior. 1-Acidophil. 2-Basophil. Cells in which cytoplasm is not conspicuous are chromophobes.

In Figure 18.2 we see the pars posterior (left) and the pars intermedia (right) of the hypophysis cerebri. The pars posterior (1) is made up of nerve fibres and neuroglial cells (details of which cannot be made out in routine sections). The pars intermedia contains some colloid filled vesicles (2), blood capillaries (3) and clumps of cells (4) in which some acidophil and basophil cells can be identified.

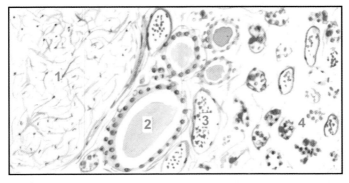

Fig. 18.2. Hypophysis cerebri. Pars posterior (left) and pars intermedia (right). 1-Pars posterior. 2-Vesicle. 3-Capillary. 4-Clumps of cells (including some acidophils and basophils).

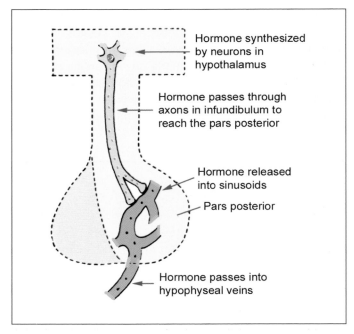

Fig. 18.3. Scheme to show the relationship of the hypothalamus and the pars posterior of the hypophysis cerebri.

The pars posterior of the hypophysis is associated with the release into the blood of two hormones. One of these is **vasopressin** (also called the **antidiuretic hormone** or ADH). This hormone controls reabsorption of water by kidney tubules. The second hormone is oxytocin. It controls the contraction of smooth muscle of the uterus and also of the mammary gland.

It is now known that these two hormones are not produced in the hypophysis cerebri at all. They are synthesized in neurons located mainly in the supraoptic and paraventricular nuclei of the hypothalamus. Vasopressin is produced mainly in the supraoptic nucleus, and oxytocin in the paraventricular nucleus. These secretions (which are bound with a glycoprotein called **neurophysin**) pass down the axons of the neurons concerned, through the infundibulum into the pars posterior. Here they are released into the capillaries of the region and enter the general circulation.

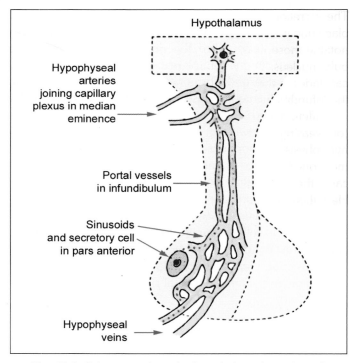

Fig. 18.4. Scheme to show the hypothalamo-hypophyseal portal circulation.

The secretion of hormones by the adenohypophysis takes place under higher control of neurons in the hypothalamus, notably those in the median eminence and in the infundibular nucleus. The axons of these neurons end in relation to capillaries in the median eminence and in the upper part of the infundibulum.

Different neurons produce specific **_releasing factors_** (or releasing hormones) for each hormone of the adenohypophysis. These factors are released into the capillaries mentioned above. Portal vessels arising from the capillaries carry these factors to the pars anterior of the hypophysis. Here they stimulate the release of appropriate hormones.

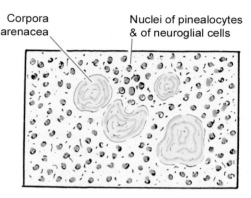

Fig. 18.5. Drawing of a section of the pineal
body as seen with a light microscope.

The pineal gland (or pineal body) is a small piriform structure
present in relation to the posterior wall of the third ventricle
of the brain. It is also called the **_epiphysis cerebri_**. The
pineal has for long been regarded as a vestigial organ of no
functional importance. (Hence the name pineal body).
However, it is now known to be an endocrine gland of great
importance.

The organ is made up mainly of cells called ***pinealocytes***. Each cell has a polyhedral body containing a spherical oval or irregular nucleus. The cell body gives off long processes with expanded ***terminal buds*** that end in relation to the wall of capillaries, or in relation to the ependyma of the third ventricle.

The pinealocytes produce a number of hormones (chemically indolamines or polypeptides). These hormones have an important regulating influence (chiefly inhibitory) on many other endocrine organs. The organs influenced include the adenohypophysis, the neurohypophysis, the thyroid, the parathyroids, the adrenal cortex and medulla, the gonads, and the pancreatic islets. The hormones of the pineal body reach the hypophysis both through the blood and through the CSF. Pineal hormones may also influence the adenohypophysis by inhibiting production of releasing factors.

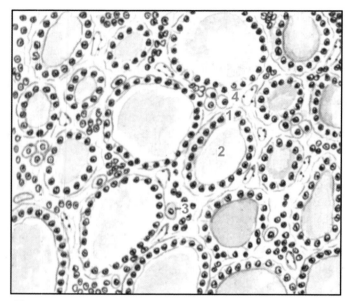

Fig. 18.6. Thyroid gland. 1-Follicle lined by cuboidal epithelium. 2-Colloid. 3-Parafollicular cells. 4-Connective tissue.

Thyroid Gland

It is made up of follicles lined by cuboidal epithelium (1). The follicles contain pink staining colloid (2). In the intervals between the follicles there is some connective tissue. Parafollicular cells (3) are present in relation to the follicles and also as groups in the connective tissue (4).

1. The follicular cells vary in shape depending on the level of their activity. Normally (at an average level of activity) the cells are cuboidal, and the colloid in the follicles is moderate in amount (Fig. 18.7).

When inactive (or resting) the cells are flat (squamous) and the follicles are distended with abundant colloid. Lastly, when the cells are highly active they become columnar and colloid is scanty. Different follicles may show differing levels of activity.

2. The follicular cells secrete two hormones that influence the rate of metabolism. Iodine is an essential constituent of these hormones. One hormone containing three atoms of iodine in each molecule is called ***triiodothyronine*** or T3. The second hormone containing four atoms of iodine in each molecule is called tetraiodothyronine, T4, or thyroxine. T3 is much more active than T4.

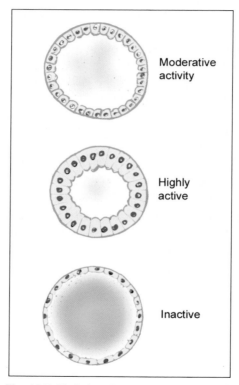

Fig. 18.7. Variations in appearance of thyroid follicles at different levels of activity.

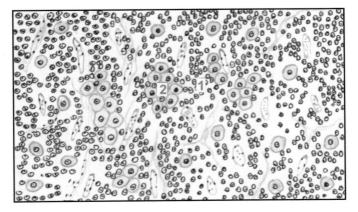

Fig. 18.8. Parathyroid gland. 1-Chief cells (only nuclei seen). 2-Oxyphil cells with pink cytoplasm. Note numerous capillaries.

Parathyroid Glands

These are made up of masses of cells with numerous capillaries in between. Most of the cells (of which only nuclei are seen) are the chief cells (1). The large cells with pink cytoplasm are oxyphil cells (2).

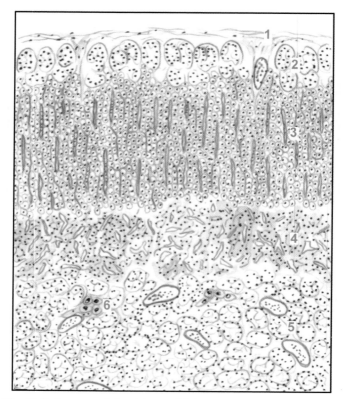

Fig. 18.9. Suprarenal gland. Upper 2/3 is cortex, lower 1/3 is medulla. 1-Capsule. 2-Zona glomerulosa. 3-Zona fasciculata. 4-Zona reticularis. 5-Medulla. 6-Sympathetic neurons.

Suprarenal Gland

Note the connective tissue capsule (1) from which septa extend into the gland substance. The gland consists of an outer cortex (upper 2/3 of figure) and an inner medulla (lower 1/3). The cortex is divisible into three zones. The zona glomerulosa (2) is most superficial. Here the cells are arranged in the form of inverted U-shaped structures or acinus-like groups. In the zona fasciculata (3) the cells are arranged in straight columns (typically two cell thick). Sinusoids intervene between the columns. The zona reticularis (4) is made up of cords of cells that branch and form a network. The medulla (5) is made up of groups of cells separated by wide sinusoids. Some sympathetic neurons (6) are also present.

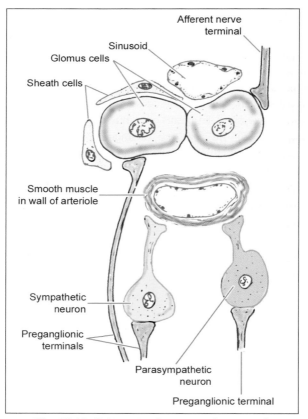

Fig. 18.10. Scheme to show some features of
the structure of the carotid body.

The Carotid Bodies

These are small oval structures, present one on each side of the neck, at the bifurcation of the common carotid artery (i.e. near the carotid sinus). The main function of the carotid bodies is that they act as chemoreceptors that monitor the oxygen and carbon dioxide levels in blood. They reflexly control the rate and depth of respiration through respiratory centres located in the brainstem. In addition to this function the carotid bodies are also believed to have an endocrine function.

The carotid bodies contain a network of capillaries in the intervals between which there are several types of cells. The carotid bodies have a rich innervation.

The most conspicuous cells of the carotid body are called **glomus cells** (or type I cells). These are large cells that have several similarities to neurons.

CHAPTER NINETEEN

The Eye

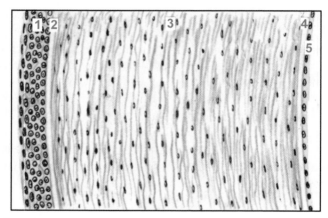

Fig. 19.1. Section through cornea. 1-Stratified squamous epithelium. 2-Anterior limiting lamina. 3-Substantia propria. 4-Posterior limiting lamina. 5-Cuboidal epithelium.

Cornea

The outermost layer (to the left)(1) is of non-keratinized stratified squamous epithelium. Next, there is the structureless anterior limiting membrane. Most of the thickness of the cornea is made up of several layers of collagen fibres embedded in a ground substance (3). These layers form the substantia propria. Deep to the substantia propria there is a thin homogeneous layer called the posterior limiting lamina (4). The posterior surface of the cornea is lined by a single layer of flattened or cuboidal cells (5).

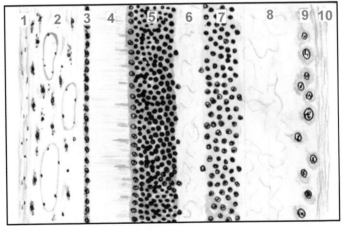

Fig. 19.2. Section through eyeball showing its layers. 3 to 10 belong to the retina. 1-Sclera. 2-Choroid. 3-Pigment cell layer. 4- Rods and cones. 5-Outer nuclear layer. 6-Outer plexiform layer. 7-Inner nuclear layer. 8-Inner plexiform layer. 9-Layer of ganglion cells. 10-Layer of optic nerve fibres.

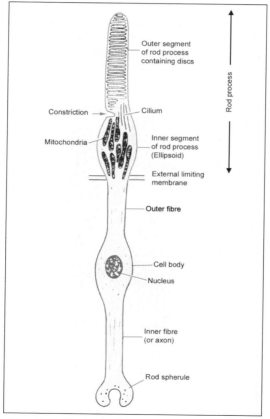

Fig. 19.3. Structure of a rod cell as seen by EM.

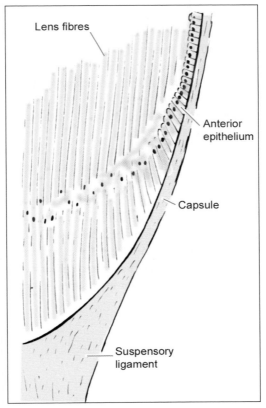

Fig. 19.4. Section through part of the lens near its margin.

Lens (See Fig. 19.4)

The surface of the lens is covered by a highly elastic lens capsule. Deep to the capsule the lens is covered on its anterior surface by a lens epithelium. The cells of the epithelium are cuboidal. However, towards the periphery of the lens the cells become progressively longer. Ultimately they are converted into long fibres that form the substance of the lens. The lens contains about 2000 such fibres.

The substance of the lens is made up of a firm inner part called the **nucleus**, and a pliable outer part the **cortex**. Both parts are made up of a number of layers or laminae. Each lamina consists of long lens fibres that are derived from the anterior epithelium. The lens fibres are made up of special transparent proteins called **crystallins**. The fibres are hexagonal in cross-section and have a regular geometric arrangement. They are attached to each other by their edges. For this purpose the edges bear knobs that fit into sockets on adjoining fibres.

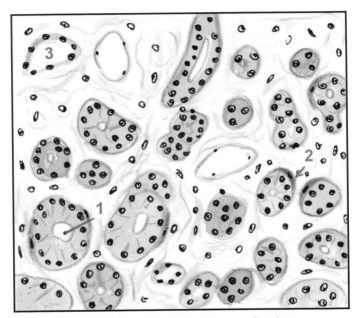

Fig. 19.5. Lacrimal gland. 1-Lumen of acinus.
2-Myoepithelial cell. 3-Duct.

Lacrimal Gland

This is a serous gland which can be distinguished by the distinct lumen of each acinus (1), and by its pink (rather than blue) staining. Myoepithelial cells (2) are present. A duct is seen at '3'.

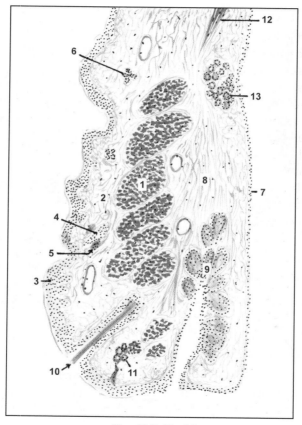

Fig. 19.6. Eyelid.

Eyelid

Like the lip the eyelid has a core of striated muscle (1) and dense connective tissue (2). Its external surface is covered by true skin (3) in which hair follicles (4), sebaceous glands (5), and sweat glands (6) are present. The inner surface is lined by palpebral conjunctiva (7): the epithelium here is stratified columnar. The connective tissue intervening between the conjunctiva and the layer of muscle is dense and forms the tarsal plate (8) in which tarsal glands (9) are embedded. An eyelash is seen at 10, just behind which there are the ciliary glands (11) which are modified sweat glands. In the upper part of the figure we see fibres of the levator palpebrae superioris (12), and accessory lacrimal glands (13).

CHAPTER TWENTY

The Ear

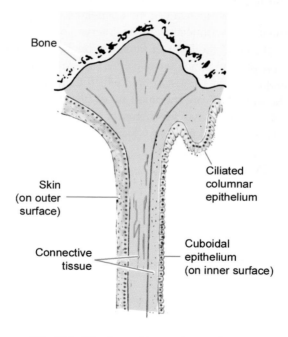

Fig. 20.1. Structure of tympanic membrane.

The Tympanic Membrane

The tympanic membrane has three layers. The middle layer is made up of fibrous tissue, which is lined on the outside by skin (continuous with that of the external acoustic meatus), and on the inside by mucous membrane of the tympanic cavity.

The fibrous layer contains collagen fibres and some elastic fibres. The fibres are arranged in two layers. In the outer layer they are placed radially, while in the inner layer they run circularly.

The mucous membrane is lined by an epithelium which may be cuboidal or squamous. It is said that the mucosa over the upper part of the tympanic membrane may have patches of ciliated columnar epithelium, but this is not borne out by EM studies.

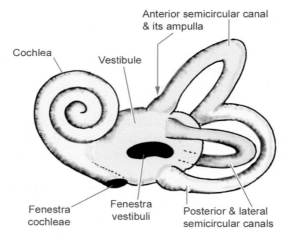

Fig. 20.2. Bony labyrinth as seen from the lateral side.

Bony Labyrinth

The bony labyrinth consists of a central part called the **vestibule**. The vestibule is continuous anteriorly with the **cochlea**; and posteriorly with three **semicircular canals**.

The cochlear part of the bony labyrinth is divisible into two parts. One part, the **scala vestibuli** opens into the vestibule; while the second part called the **scala tympani** opens into the middle ear through an aperture called the **fenestra cochleae.**

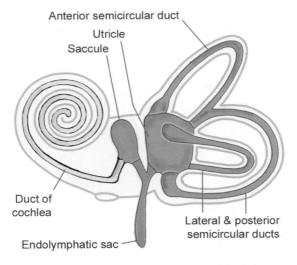

Anterior semicircular duct
Utricle
Saccule
Duct of cochlea
Endolymphatic sac
Lateral & posterior semicircular ducts

Fig. 20.3. Parts of the membranous labyrinth.

Membranous Labyrinth

The parts of the membranous labyrinth are shown in Figure 20.3. Within each semicircular canal the membranous labyrinth is represented by a **semicircular duct**. The part of the membranous labyrinth present in the cochlea is called the **duct of the cochlea**. The part of the membranous labyrinth that lies within the vestibule is in the form of two distinct membranous sacs called the **saccule** and the **utricle**.

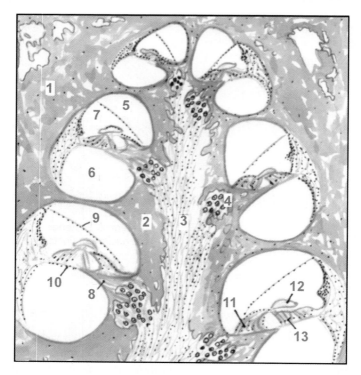

Fig. 20.4. Cochlea (low power view). 1-Petrous temporal bone. 2-Modiolus. 3-Canal for passage of cochlear nerve fibres. 4-Spiral ganglion. 5-Scala vestibuli. 6-Scala tympani. 7-Duct of cochlea. 8-Spiral lamina. 9-Vestibular membrane. 10-Basilar membrane. 11-Spiral limbus. 12-Membrana tectoria. 13-Organ of Corti.

Cochlea

This is a low power view to show the general structure of the cochlea.

The cochlea is embedded in the petrous temporal bone (1). It is in the form of a spiral canal and is, therefore, cut up six times. The cone-shaped mass of bone surrounded by these turns of the cochlea is called the modiolus (2) which contains a canal through which fibres of the cochlear nerve (3) pass. A mass of neurons belonging to the spiral ganglion (4) lies to the inner side of each turn of the cochlea.

The parts to be identified in each turn of the cochlea are the scala vestibuli (5), the scala tympani (6), the duct of the cochlea (7), the spiral lamina (8), the vestibular membrane (9), the basilar membrane (10), the spiral limbus (11), the membrana tectoria (12), and the organ of Corti (13).

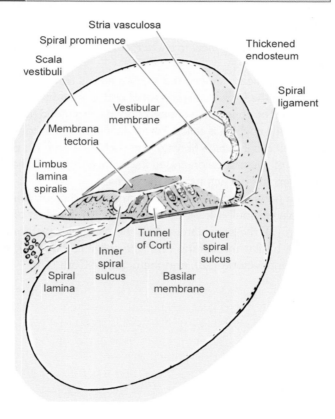

Fig. 20.5. Section across one turn of the cochlea to show some of its features.

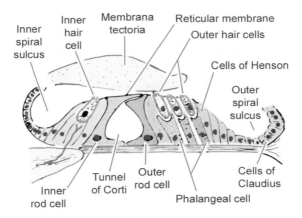

Fig. 20.6. Diagram to show the cells in the organ of Corti.

The Spiral Organ of Corti

The spiral organ of Corti is so called because (like other structures in the cochlea) it extends in a spiral manner through the turns of the cochlea. In sections it is seen to be placed on the basilar membrane and to be made up of epithelial cells that are arranged in a complicated manner. The cells are divisible into the true receptor cells or **hair cells**, and supporting elements which are given different names depending on their location. The cells of the spiral organ are covered from above by a gelatinous mass called the **membrana tectoria**.

Index